Diagnostic Skills in Chinese Medicine

Book 1: The Four Diagnostic Skills

By Cat Calhoun, MAcOM, L.Ac.

Cats TCM Notes Press
San Miguel de Allende, Mexico

*For DeLora, my sunshine and my flowers.
Thank you with all my heart for your supporting
and for sticking with me through Chinese Medicine School!*

This page intentionally left blank

ACKNOWLEDGMENTS

No one does anything truly on their own. I thought myself totally self-sufficient before I dove into the study of Chinese medicine. When that journey began, my eyes opened to the myriads of those who were actively helping me, those who have gone before, and even those who will come long after I'm gone. We are interconnected. You are me, I am you.

I especially want to thank Dr. Song Luo, my teacher and coolest clinical supervisors I had. Such kindness, compassion and wisdom! Thank you for your patience and guidance.

Thank you to Lisa Lapwing, a most awesome practitioner based in Orlando Florida. We studied together, practiced together, we practiced *on* each other in student clinic, and then we became each others' practitioners! Not having Lisa in my daily life is my one giant regret about moving to Mexico.

Thank you to my buds: Donna "Needles" Tatum, Tiffany Chiu Peralez, Vanessa Olsen, Andi Kohn, Mark Hernandez, and Katherine Webster. To Georgie Hoiseth, a kick ass practitioner and fellow computer geek, I thank thee! To Rita Ramirez, I would *NOT* want to be on this journey without you!

To my patients, whom I learn from every day and who trust me with their healthcare, thank you. I love having you in my life.

And to so many more who have loved, supported, and believed in me, I express my gratitude and thanks. May the deity of your choice look favorably upon you all!

Cat Calhoun

ACKNOWLEDGMENTS	5
Chapter 1	*11*
Section 1: Observation and Inspection	**13**
Chapter 2: Observing the Shen	*15*
Chapter 3: Classifying the Body	*17*
Yin and Yang Body Type Classification	17
Excess Yang or Yang Abundant Body Type	17
Excess Yin or Yin Abundant Body Type	18
Yang Deficient Body Type	19
Yin Deficient Body Type.	19
Five Element Body Classification	20
Body Build Types	22
Chapter 4: Observing the Complexion	*23*
"Normal" Color	23
Dominant Color	24
Guest Color	24
Pathological Color	25
Conforming and Opposing Color	26
Individual Color Pathology Analysis	26
White/Pale Complexions	26
Sallow complexion color	27
Yellow complexion colors	27
Red complexion coloration	28
Blue/Green complexions	28
Dark complexions	29
Purple complexion colors	30
How emotions affect coloring	30
Chapter 5: Observing the Body	*31*
Observation of Body Movements	31
Tremors of the head	32
Rigidity of the neck	33
Deviation of the eyes and mouth	34
Limbs and body	36
Observation of the Head, Face, and Hair	37
What to look or on the head	37
Facial s/sx	37
Hair observations	38
Observation of the Eyes – Five Wheel Diagnosis	40
Observation of the Nose	42
Observation of Philtrum, Lips and Mouth, Teeth & Gums	44

Philtrum	44
Lips and Mouth	44
Teeth and Gums	44
Observation of the Ears	46
Observations of the Nails	47
Observations of Chest/Abdomen	48
Observation of the Four Limbs	48
Observation of Body Secretions	49
Observation of the Skin	50
Observation of the Abdomen	51
Observation of Children	52
Chapter 6: Tongue Diagnosis	*55*
Preparation	55
Lighting	55
Medications	56
Foods and Drinks	56
Tongue scraping	56
How to Look at the Tongue	57
Have your patient stick their tongue out	57
Normal Tongue Presentation	58
Pathological Tongue Body Presentation	58
Tongue body colors	58
Tongue body shape and other anomalies	60
Tongue body movement	61
Pathological Tongue Coatings	61
Section 2: Listening and Smelling	**65**
Chapter 7: Listening	*67*
Listening to the Voice	67
Abnormal Language	68
Listening to Respiration	69
Coughing	70
Digestive Noises	71
Vomiting	71
Hiccups	71
Chapter 8: Smelling	*73*
Belching Smells	73
Rotten Apple Smell	73
Other Disturbing Smells	74
Section 3: Asking Questions	**75**

Chapter 9: The Ten Traditional Questions	*77*
The Basics of Interviewing	78
Getting a Full History	80
The Chief Complaint	80
Present History	81
Past History	82
Personal History	82
Family History	83
The Ten Traditional Questions	83
1. Aversion to chills, fever	83
2. Sweating	85
3. Head and Body	87
4. Urine and Stool	90
5. Eating and Drinking	94
6. Chest and Abdomen Questions	97
7. Hearing and deafness	98
Questions 8, 9, and 10	99
Chapter 10: The Sixteen Modern Questions	*101*
Taste	101
Energy Level	102
Sleep	103
Diseases Specific to Women	106
Emotional Symptoms	108
Section 4: Pulse Diagnosis	**111**
Chapter 11: Pulse Diagnosis Basics	*113*
Pulse Diagnosis Introduction	113
The uber-basics	114
Pulse Basics – Beyond Uber-basics	115
The pulse points	116
What the positions represent on either side	116
Finding the pulse points	117
How long to take the pulse	119
How deep to press	120
Best time to take the pulse	120
Ideal posture	120
Method for pulse taking	121
An ideal pulse	122
How fast should the pulse be?	123
Chapter 12: Pathological Pulses	*125*
Superficial Pulses	125

Deep Pulses	129
Slow Pulses	132
Rapid Pulses	134
Deficient Pulses	136
Excess Pulses	138
A quick chat about "Slippery"	142
Strange and Death Pulses	143
Section 4: Palpation	**145**
Chapter 13: Palpation	*147*
Palpating Skin and Muscle	147
Palpating Hands and Feet	148
Palpating the Chest and Abdomen	149
Apical pulse	149
Palpating the Chest/Hypochrondria	150
Abdominal Palpation and Pain	150
Biomedical categorizations about abdominal pain	150
Chinese medical categorizations about abdominal pain and palpation	151
Bonus Section: Study Questions and Answers	*153*
About the author	*203*

CHAPTER 1
Introduction to Chinese Medical Diagnostics

Chinese Medicine is the Sherlock Holmes of medical models. Everything is important, all the clues are considered, then a diagnosis is crafted by assembling what we know. There are four critical diagnostic skills used:

Observation and Inspection	Observing the exterior of the body with your own eyes to determine the patient's condition of illness or health.
Listening and Smelling	Listening to the sounds this patient's body makes – breathing and coughing sounds, vocal quality, intestinal sounds, for example.
Asking Questions	Interviewing the patient
Palpation	Feeling pulse quality, but also palpating the channels and the body

Chinese medicine authors say that what happens inside the body will manifest externally in visible signs and symptoms. Observation is about looking, listening, and paying attention to what you discover.

In Chinese medicine we don't open up the patient to see what's inside, we make extremely informed guess based on observation in a forensic way.

To do a good Chinese medicine diagnosis you use the four basic skills as well diagnostic models such as the Eight Principles, Zangfu Diagnosis, the Six Stages, the Four Levels, and meridian and channel theory diagnosis. Be aware that there are a number of other diagnostic models you could use for crafting a diagnosis and treatment plan.

This book will cover in some depth the four basic skills. Book 2 covers the diagnostic models.

SECTION 1:
OBSERVATION AND INSPECTION

Observation and inspection of the outside of the body will give you many windows into what is happening on the inside of the body. In Chinese medicine we observe the Shen, the exterior of the body for constitutional type, the complexion, body movements, the eyes, and the tongue.

This page intentionally left blank.

Chapter 2
Observing the Shen

There are three aspects of spirit or Shen. There is the embodiment, which is the outward manifestation of a person's spirit within the body. There is vitality, a reflection of a person's energy. And finally, there is luster. In the west we say the eyes are the windows of the soul. A similar saying in China is "the eyes are the window of the spirit." The luster of the spirit shines in a person's eyes. If the Shen of a person is strong, their prognosis will be better than the prognosis of a person whose Shen is weakened.

Strong Shen characterizes a strong spirit. A strong Shen will show in the body in this way:

Strong Shen	Presentation
Eyes	Sparkling, clear eyes
Face	Lively expression with a lustrous complexion
Mental/emotional state	• Clear and alert mind • Enthusiastic • High spirits • Positive approach to life • Stable personality • Strong will power • Clear sense of direction in life • Keen intellect
Other physical aspects	• Good reflexes • Good energy • Normal breathing • Clear voice • Agile body movements

Now compare this to someone who has a *weak* Shen.

Weak Shen	Presentation
Eyes	Dull, no sparkle
Face	Lusterless complexion
Tongue	Without spirit. . . what? Yeah, my professor really said that. He said "you'll know." I still don't. All I got out of him was "Possible heart crack in the tongue."
Mental/emotional state	• Listlessness • Lack of enthusiasm • Confused thinking • May suffer from apathy • Depression • Lack of willpower • Confusion about their path in life • Slow intellect
Other physical aspects	• Shallow breathing • Weak voice • Slow body movements

One final aspect of Shen you should be aware of is that of "false shen." False shen only appears during the course of a severe chronic disease. The patient will suddenly present with the appearance of vigor and health, but this is not true. This is like the last radiance of the sun before it sets. It is a surge of Yang as it is separating from the Yin of the body. This surge gives the Qi temporary vigor before death.

False Shen looks like this:
- Sudden onset of vigor
- Clear look in the eyes
- Talking more, maybe incessantly
- Wants to meet with family
- Improvement of appetite
- Complexion is pinker, but upon closer in section the color seems to be sitting on the surface like paint rather than coming from inside the body.

CHAPTER 3
Classification of the Body

There are numerous books on body types and how that affects health. If you walk through a book store and don't see at least a few, then you're not walking through the health section! Chinese medicine also classifies body types in an effort to help understand health, potential health challenges, and predispositions.

There are five different ways in which we classify body type:
- Yin and Yang classification
- Five Element classification
- Classification according to prenatal and postnatal influences
- Body build classification
- Classification by pain and drug tolerance

We will take a closer look at three of these ways: Yin and Yang, Five Element, and body build.

YIN AND YANG BODY TYPE CLASSIFICATION
This should remind you of the Yin and Yang excesses you studied in Chapter 2 of *Chinese Medicine 101: Start with the Foundations* (ISBN: 1093826703). Bodies here are classified by these parameters, as you will see.

Excess Yang or Yang Abundant Body Type
Yang is strongly tied to Qi. An abundance of Yang brings an abundance of heat signs and symptoms, but also an abundance of energy.

Body Component	Presentation
Face	Tendency for the face to be red
Temperature	• Preference for cold • Preference for light clothing • Intolerance to heat
Body/Physical demeanor	• Strong body build • Loud voice • Tends to walk with chest and stomach projecting forward.
Emotional demeanor	• Lively character • High achiever • Active • Talkative in nature • Tendency to laugh

Excess Yin or Yin Abundant Body Type

Yin abundance is tied to Blood and body fluids and a tendency toward cold.

Body Component	Presentation
Face	Relatively dark complexion
Temperature	• Preference for heat • Desire to wrap up warmly • Preference for summer season and warmth
Body/Physical demeanor	• Tendency towards obesity • Loose muscle tone with thick skin
Emotional demeanor	• Quiet • Reticent • Introverted

Yang Deficient Body Type

Here you see a low spirit with no fire or energy. This is because Yang and Qi are so closely intertwined – without strong Yang, there is weak Qi. Yang is weak and yin looks relatively strong by comparison. This is commonly seen in clinic – overweight, pale and bluish.

Body Component	Presentation
Face	Pale or pale bluish complexion
Temperature	• Preference for warmth • Aversion to cold • Cold limbs • Desire to wrap up
Body/Physical demeanor	• Overweight or swollen body • Weak, loose muscles • Slow movement
Emotional demeanor	• Low spirit. No fire or energy because of the weak Yang

Yin Deficient Body Type.

This leaves Yang as the comparatively stronger force in the body. Note the less avid presentations of Yang here than you see in the Yang abundant type. The occasional red cheeks and lips are an expression of Yang surfacing because it is not grounded by sufficient Yin.

Body Component	Presentation
Face	• Red cheeks, but only zygomatic area • Red lips (sometimes) • Restless expression in the eyes
Temperature	• Feelings of heat
Body/Physical demeanor	• Thin body • Tall • Long shaped head

	• Narrow shoulders • Long and flat chest • Quick movements • Walks or stands bent forward
Emotional demeanor	• Looks excited • Tends to *be* excited

FIVE ELEMENT BODY CLASSIFICATION

Unless this is the first book on Chinese medicine you've ever picked up, this won't shock you: Five Element Body Classification is based on the five elements. What's the point of this? When you classify someone correctly, you can use the Five Element theories to understand their health problems, how they arose, and what they are likely to face if they stay on their current track.

I'll lay this out for you in a chart. **If it's bold, pay attention.** These are considered definitive and strong characteristics for the type. Unfortunately, when you're publishing notes like this you only get a certain amount of real estate on the page, whether it's digital or printed. I've got some notes for you on this chart, but look it over first and then read the notes.

	Wood	Fire	Earth	Metal	Water
Cmplx Color	Green	Red	Yellow	Pale	Dark
Head	Small	Pointed/small	Large	Small	Large
Face	Long		Round	Square	
Teeth		Wide			
Jaw			Wide		Broad cheeks
Shoulder	Broad	Well dev'd	Well dev'd	Small	Narrow
Voice				**Strong**	
Back	Straight		Well dev'd		
Abdomen			Large	Flat	Large

Heart/vessels		**Strong**			
Sinew	**Ropy/ sinewy**				
Height	Tall				
Walk/gait			Brisk	Slow	
Muscle			**Strong**		Long spine
Kidneys					**Strong**

Those notes I promised:

- Cmplx Color is *Complexion* Color. These aren't Teletubbies we are treating, so this is the undertone hue to the face. We *all* have this, regardless of race.

- Head and Face both refer to the overall shape of the head or face.

- Teeth . . . Wide? Not really sure I've seen what I would call "wide" teeth. Maybe this refers to a wide smile.

- "Well dev'd" means well developed in Cat Abbreviation Land.

- Heart/Vessels refers to pulse mostly. Strong pulse with a healthy feeling vessel. Can also be a strong heart beat when you listen with a stethoscope.

- "Ropy/sinewy" looking body. Not necessarily pumped and cut, but you they have a ropy, sinewy body look.

- Strong Kidneys – you'll know this after you do your intake with them.

Body Build Types

I mention this because it is culturally dependent, so this is relative to your and your patient's culture. The Thin and Overweight types are really the most clinically relevant for you.

Type	Tendency
Robust	Yang excess
Compact	Smooth circulation of Qi and Blood. Tend to suffer deficiency of Qi and Blood.
Muscular	Qi and Blood are strong and Middle Jiao will transform Qi and Blood easily.
Thin	Qi and Blood deficiency, sometimes Yin deficiency
Overweight	Qi deficiency, especially of the Middle Jiao, so will also tend toward damp retention. And probably phlegm too.

CHAPTER 4
Observing the Complexion

Your goal here is to be able to spot normal and pathological skin complexion colors. That's your *goal*. Are you going to be able to do that after one class or after reading these notes? Nope. But the more you practice this the better you'll get. This is a learned skill.

To build your chops:
>Train yourself to look at the color or people's complexions as you walk by them, sit next to them while you study, etc. Don't try to analyze this with your brain cells. Just notice and let it go.
>
>>Hint: if you're having a hard time with this, look at the color at the temples. It's often more obvious and changes more readily than in other places. Also seems to show a truer color.
>
>And please don't stare. We don't need people thinking acupuncturists are creepers!

"Normal" Color

Before you can spot a counterfeit $20 bill, you first have to know exactly what a real bill looks like. The same is true in looking at the complexion. Fortunately, we've all grown up as humans (I know you could probably make an argument against this in some cases), so we know what faces look like and we can all probably glance at a person who isn't healthy and know that something is off.

What you're looking at in the facial complexion is the health of the Qi and Blood. When both of these are flourishing and flowing well, the complexion has luster, the skin has moisture, and the person seems to glow a bit. Here is how my professor defined 'normal.'

> *Normal refers to luster and hue or coloring of the complexion. If there is luster, the complexion is shining, reflecting a strong Qi. A subtle reddish hue means the blood is not deficient. This is **inside** of the skin and shines out, indicating that Yin and Yang are in harmony. Sufficient moisture to the skin indicates there is no deficiency or harm to the Body Fluids.*
>
> --Dr. Song Luo

Dominant Color

Dominant color is what you were born with before any environmental or life factors started shifting this color.

Do you remember the people "having their colors done?" It's still kind of a thing. This was a color analysis to find your native skin tones and coloring and then pinpoint what colors you could wear that made you look amazing. This is kind of what I'm talking about.

Everyone has a basic underlying skin tone and hue and that is normal. It is determined by race and prenatal factors and it relates to your body type.

Guest Color

Guest color is coloring you take on as a result of physiological, seasonal, climatic, geographic and working conditions change the coloring. Kind of like working at the neighborhood pool for the summer and getting a tan.

A person with a wood type, for example, would have a dominant underlying color that is greenish. In the summer the color might look a little more red. If this person had a Liver fire problem, their pathological coloring would be a deep red.

PATHOLOGICAL COLOR

Complexions change all time, even in a completely healthy person, because as the experiences and emotions flow through life it has a small impact in Qi and Blood and that shows in the face. When we get angry there is a slight bluish tint that colors the face, more red when we are really happy, blackish when we are afraid, etc. That's not pathology, that's just life.

Pathological color sticks around regardless of the current emotional landscape. You'll see it throughout your time with the patient and it reflects an imbalance or imbalances in the body.

Here are some basic characteristics, pairs of opposites, to be aware of in regard to pathological coloring.

Characteristic	Meaning
Superficial	Condition is mild, on the exterior, or Yang
Deep	Condition is severe, in the interior, or Yin
Distinct	Yang type of disease, superficial, Upright Qi is not exhausted
Obscure	Yin type of disease, deep, Upright Qi is weakened
Scattered*	Mild disease, short in duration, weak pathogen. Prognosis is good.
Concentrated*	Severe disease, long in duration, strong pathogen. Prognosis is not so good.
Thin	Like a single coat of thin paint. Deficiency or acute disease
Thick	Thick paint – several coats Excess or chronic disease
Luster*	Good spirit, weak pathogenic factors, mild condition. Prognosis is good.
Lusterless*	Spirit is weak, pathogens are strong, severe condition. Prognosis is not good.

*Note the ones that reflect prognosis.

Conforming and Opposing Color

The idea of conforming and opposing color is based on the five element theory.

First, determine the dominant color of the person. Next, look at the color they are displaying and put it into the Five Element chart. Mother/Son relationship colors in relation to dominant color is pretty good. If you see a controlling or rebelling color,

Coloring	Meaning	Prognosis
Mother color	Conforming to Five Element flow.	OK
Son color	Slightly opposing.	Not bad
Overcontrolling Element color	Opposing	Worse
Insulting color	Strongly opposing	Awful

INDIVIDUAL COLOR PATHOLOGY ANALYSIS

This is a breakdown of the individual colors that can show in the complexion and how to interpret them. Pay attention to the **bold** below. Those are pretty definitive.

White/Pale Complexions

White coloration indicates deficiency or cold. Pale indicates either cold or a lack of nourishment.

Color	Interpretation
Bright white	**Yang** deficiency of Middle Jiao, Lu, Ht, Ki. Less Yang to warm the body gives this color. Qi and blood deficiency can lead to the paleness.
Dull white	More severe Yang deficiency than above.
Pale white	**Qi deficiency**. Pale face, specifically
Sallowy white*	**Blood deficiency**
Bluish white	Cold, especially from Yang deficiency

*See more on sallow complexions below.
Note: Yin deficiency will not be pale every because lack of Yin = relatively too much Yang, which gives a redder color, but only on the zygomatic areas. If the whole cheek is red, then it's more likely to be a Yang excess.

Sallow complexion color

Sallow is a pale/yellowish color rather than a white complexion. This complexion is dull and without luster, indicating a deficiency and/or dampness. Dampness is so sticky it even grabs the color of the complexion, holding it inside and causing the lusterless look. **Pay attention to the bolded stuff.**

Color	Interpretation
Sallow	**Spleen Qi deficiency and/or dampness**
	Could also be a Kidney Yang deficiency
Sallow/grey	Sallow as indicated above + grey which is Blood stasis. I've always thought of this as "heart patient grey."

Yellow complexion colors

Indicates deficiency (usually Spleen Qi xu) and/or dampness. Pay specific attention to the **bolded** stuff below.

Color	Interpretation
Pale yellow	Spleen Qi deficiency, blood deficiency, anemia
Grayish yellow	Spleen Qi deficiency with stagnation of Lv Qi or Blood
Yellow and dry	Full or empty heat in St and Sp, indicating that heat is strong and burning the Body Fluids
Ash-like yellow	Dampness
Bright yellow	**Damp and heat – this is jaundice**
Dark yellow	**Damp and cold – this is another form of jaundice**

Red complexion coloration

Red indicates heat. Pay attention to *where* the red is on the body and to the description.

Color	Interpretation
Red cheeks	Full/excess heat due to Yang excess affecting Ht, Lu, Lv, or St. High fever can be one reason for this.
Whole face red	
Red cheekbones	Red zygomatic region only is due to empty heat caused by Yin deficiency of Lu, Ht, St, or Ki. Can also be blood deficiency.
Floating red	Empty heat or false heat/true cold

Blue/Green complexions

Blue/Green colorations indicate cold, pain, blood stasis, or inner wind. Generally speaking, this is *due to an excess* of one or more of those conditions, but it is *not associated with deficiency*. It is also *not* associated with damp, which has a yellow type color.

The coloring is due to the impediment or blockage of the circulation of Qi and/or blood, constrictions of the meridian/s and blood stasis. All of those are about congestion and stagnation. I associate this with bruises resulting from trauma. This too is a form of stasis and can help you remember this.

You don't need to memorize this in detail unless your instructor tells you to, but you do need to know those basic concepts above.

Color	Interpretation
Pale blue under eyes	Lv Qi stagnation
Dark bluish under eyes	Cold in Lv channel
White/bluish	Cold or chronic pain

Bluish in kids	Lv wind
Green with red tinge	Lesser Yang syndrome
Green with red eyes	Lv fire
Yellowish green cheeks	Phlegm with Lv Yang
Green nose	Qi stagnation with pain in the abdomen
Dark reddish-green	Stagnation of Lv Qi turning to heat
Grass-like green	Collapse of Lv Qi.

Dark complexions

According to the Five Element Theory, dark/black is related to the Kidney. This type of complexion coloring is attributed to Kidney deficiency, long term cold conditions, Blood stasis, and/or phlegm-fluid retention. At the beginning, cold presents as pale, but long term becomes purple or bluish.

Color	Interpretation
Dark and dry	Ki Yin deficiency
Dull, dark	Ki Yang deficiency with internal cold
Dark around eye socket	Ki deficiency with phlegm fluids or cold damp in Lower Jiao
Dull, dark	Like soot. Damp cold and/or phlegm fluid retention
Faintly dark	Damp cold or phlegm fluid retention
Very dark	Blood stasis

Purple complexion colors

This is really a deeper version of bluish or greenish coloration and indicates stasis.

Color	Interpretation
Reddish purple	Blood stasis
Bluish purple	Internal cold leading to Blood stasis....or poisoning. Wasn't that a medieval moment?

Changes of purple coloration can occur due to blood stasis. It starts as a dark blue purple, changing to greenish, then to yellowish.

HOW EMOTIONS AFFECT COLORING

Emotions can affect the complexion. Check this out.

Color	Interpretation
Anger	Green on cheeks, under eyes
Mania	In CM speak, "excessive joy" Reddish tint to complexion
Worry	Grayish, without luster
Pensiveness	Sallow yellow
Fear	Bright white on cheeks and forehead
Shock	Bright whitish blue
Hatred	Dull greenish, without luster
Craving	Reddish on cheeks
Guilt	Dark, ruddy

CHAPTER 5
Observing the Body

Because Chinese medicine is a Sherlock Holmes hunt for clues, let's continue the study with the movements of the body, observations about the head, face, and hair, the eyes, nose, mouth, ears, nails, and more.

This chapter contains Five Wheel diagnosis (eye diagnosis) and diagnosis of children, all of which will come up on several tests, including the national boards if you are in the United States. (If you're looking for tongue diagnosis, that's the following chapter.)

OBSERVATION OF BODY MOVEMENTS

Mostly, this is about looking for manifestations of wind. It presents in many ways, but it always comes down to Liver. My professors were fond of throwing Chinese phrases at us, so I'm going to pass this hot potato on to you:

> Zhu feng diao xuan jie shu yu gan.
>
> *Different wind (zhu feng) uncontrollable (diao) circling/vertigo/dizziness (xuan) are all related to Liver.*

Liver, per the Five Element Theory, is related to wind. Tremors are caused by wind, regardless of whether it is inner wind or exterior wind. Another manifestation of wind in the body is paralysis or hemiplegia.

Bell's Palsy is a good example of hemiplegia caused by external wind. External wind is caused by external conditions. In the case of Bell's Palsy, it is a literal exterior wind that invades the body and creates the right conditions for Bell's to manifest.

Inner wind, conversely, is not caused by external forces, but has endogenous causes. Inner wind includes presentations such as epilepsy and Parkinson's Disease. Hypertension can *cause* Inner wind.

You can see Liver Wind in a red, angry face or in dizziness or in hemiplegia and paralysis.

The two main reasons inner wind occurs in the body are extreme heat and blood deficiency.

Inner wind cause	Brief discussion
Extreme heat	Heat generates wind in the environment and in us. Anger is one form. Chronic depression can lead to fire due to long term Liver Qi stagnation. Look for a red face, dizziness, vertigo.
Blood deficiency	Perhaps from chronic malnutrition. Blood is insufficient, thus does not carry the Qi or flow properly and gets stagnant. Stagnation leads to heat which leads to wind. Can also manifest as itchiness on the skin, another form of wind. Like wind, those s/sx can come and go quickly.

Tremors of the head

This is probably the most important sign of wind in the body.

Look or shaking of the head, *usually* back and forth. Tremor can range from very light w/ small amplitude to pronounced with large amplitude

- Mild tremors: deficiency.
  Generally lasts longer and is more chronic

- More severe tremors: excess
  Usually of short duration and more acute

You will see two types of tremors:

Type	Brief discussion
Full/excess	Lv Fire or Lv Yang rising Too much heat in the body
Empty/deficient	Lv and Ki Yin deficiency or Lv Blood deficiency Lv and Ki Yin xu is the more common of the two. When Yin is deficient, Yang is relatively too strong, and is not balanced by Yin. This produces heat, which produces wind…just like in the environment when heat leads to tornados and hurricanes. Yang Qi is very light an easily floats upward. Hypertension is linked to the deficient type

Rigidity of the neck

Neck rigidity can result from sleeping weirdly or from wind exposure, both resulting in pain and stiffness.

Please note that this doesn't apply to neck stiffness due to trauma. That is trauma leading to a localized Qi and blood stagnation.

Some things you would ask in a clinical situation if a person came in with this:

Question	Brief discussion
Where is the location of the pain?	Have the patient point to the exact location. Way more effective than verbal descriptions
How long has it lasted?	Acute problems are 21 days or less. Chronic problems are longer in duration. The more chronic it becomes, the more this points to a deficient condition.
Ask what makes it better or worse	Always good to know what they have tried.
Is the pain fixed or moving?	Fixed: it's probably stasis Moving: it's probably wind-related
What is the nature of the pain?	In addition to strong, mild, fixed, and moving, this can tell you a lot: • Neck stiffness with aversion to wind and a floating pulse: External wind invasion • Neck stiffness and pain: Cold damp invasion • Slight rigidity + dizziness: Bl and Ki deficiency

Deviation of the eyes and mouth

You're looking for signs of paralysis, basically. In both central and peripheral nervous system paralysis you will see a difference between one side of the face and the other. The mouth and eye will seem to droop down on one side, the ability to wrinkle the forehead might disappear on one side, and the nasolabial groove will disappear on one side.

How to determine the healthy side:

Facial feature	Brief discussion
Mouth	Mouth is pulled toward the healthy side Because the muscles still work on the healthy side.
Nasolabial groove	Still has a visible crease
Forehead	Can wrinkle and move forehead on the healthy side

How to determine the affected side

Facial feature	Brief discussion
Mouth	Droops down on affected side. May drool from this side. Cannot smile, grimace, or bulge cheeks on this side. Can chew, but cannot get food out of this side.
Nasolabial groove	Extremely shallow or not present. Muscles are slack.
Forehead	In a peripheral nervous system problem, inability to wrinkle forehead on affected side.*
Eye	In a peripheral nervous system problem, cannot completely close the eye on the affected side. This eye will leak and may turn upward.

*That pesky forehead wrinkle.
If you read back through the intro paragraph the forehead wrinkle is the only one I said "might" on. Why?

Because there are two types of paralysis: central nervous system and peripheral nervous system.

- Peripheral (PNS) facial paralysis
  In this type of paralysis the patient *loses the ability to wrinkle the forehead* on the affected side. If this patient has longstanding wrinkles on the forehead, those will smooth out on the affected side.

Waaay better prognosis on this type. This affects the peripheral nervous tissue, which can probably recover more easily than the brain related kind below. This is usually a case of Bell's Palsy.

- Central (CNS) facial paralysis
  This is from a stroke in the cerebral tissue, so you will probably see more than just the face affected. In this type of paralysis the patient *still has forehead wrinkles and can move both sides of the forehead.* The eyes will also be OK in this type, but the mouth will be affected.

Limbs and body

This is also about tremors, which is an inability to control the limb/s. . . and it's still a presentation of wind. A short laundry list of what this includes and is still wind:

- Paralysis
- Tremor or spasticity of limbs
- Twitching of muscles
- Opisthotonos
  Spine and neck curve backwards and spasm
- Contraction of limbs
- Hemiplegia
- Tremor of hands
- Tremor of feet
- Restless leg syndromes
- Contraction of fingers

Observation of the Head, Face, and Hair

What to look or on the head

Feature/s/sx	Interpretation
Dry scalp	Lv and/or Ki Yin deficiency
Red and painful scalp	Wind heat or Lv fire
Head tremors	Lv wind
Swelling of head and face	Wind heat
Boils and ulcer	Full heat or toxic heat
Head leaning to one side	Spleen or marrow deficiency
Head tilted with eyes rolled up	Lv wind
Late closure of fontanelles	Both should be closed at around 18 months. Posterior fontanel should lose by 4 months. If this doesn't happen, Ki Essence deficiency is the likely candidate.

Facial s/sx

Feature/s/sx	Interpretation
Acute edema	Wind and water in the Lu
Chronic edema	Lu and/or Sp Yang deficiency. Should be pale in color
Acute swelling and redness	Wind toxic heat
Ulcers under zygomatic arch	Toxic heat in St
Papules on face or nose	Lu heat at the Qi level
Macules on face or nose	Blood heat
Lined face with uneven skin surface	Blood deficient heat and dryness
Deviation of the eye and mouth	Wind syndrome. See above.

Hair observations

There are several problems relating to hair to understand.

Hair falling out

Hair falling out is a blood disorder, regardless of the cause. Make a note! It's in **bold!**

Usually, it's a Lv Blood problem, but not always. Here are some likely possible causes:
- Lv Blood/Kd Essence deficiencies
- Blood heat from Lv fire
- Serious, acute disease
- Chronic, protracted disease
- Chemotherapy or radiation
- Extreme stress

Alopecia

Alopecia is when the hair rather suddenly starts falling out in clumps. This is related to wind and to Blood xu (deficiency). Any internal wind or Blood heat can cause this. Look for these manifestations with an alopecia patient.

Manifestation	Interpretation
Blood heat	Hair falls out in clumps
Internal wind	Giddiness with a wiry pulse
Blood stasis	Dark complexion with a purple tongue

Dry, brittle hair

This is caused by either Blood deficiency or Yin deficiency. This likely arose from:
- Lv Blood deficiency or Ki Essence deficiency
- General Qi and Blood deficiency
- St/Sp deficiency
- Chronic loss of blood

Greasy hair
Depending on where you live, this could just be a hipster thing! But if you discover during the intake that this is problematic or common and they actually do wash their hair regularly, it's likely they have other signs pointing to:
- Dampness or phlegm

Premature graying of hair
Four basic causes here:
- Lv Blood and/or Ki Essence deficiency
- General Qi and Blood deficiency
- Lv and Ht fire
- Hereditary disorder

Dandruff
Dandruff is caused by wind, deficiency, or excess. The top candidates are:
- Lv Blood deficiency
- Lv Wind
- Lv Fire
- Damp heat in Lv
- Toxic heat

OBSERVATION OF THE EYES – FIVE WHEEL DIAGNOSIS

Observation of the eyes is very important, since the eyes really are the windows to the soul. Mental condition can be observed through the eyes. And so can a bunch of other things. This is called *Five Wheel Diagnosis* and you'll see it frequently on diagnostics tests and on national boards.

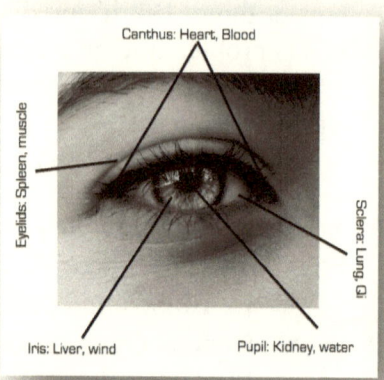

Five Wheel Diagnosis is based on Five Element Theory. Each component of the eye can reflect the health or imbalance of the body and the associations are very Five Element oriented.

I gave you some five element associations for each of the components in Five Wheel Diagnosis…except for the eyelid/Spleen association. Unless you are wearing yellow eyeshadow, that association doesn't really work here. But the rest do, so yay.

Part of the eye	Interpretation
Eyelids	Spleen and Muscle The appearance of the eyelids reflects the health of the Spleen and muscle tissues.
Canthi	Heart and Blood The inner and outer canthus should be red or pink. Red is the color associated with heart and fire in the Five Element chart.
Sclera	Lung and Qi The white part of the eye should be clear and not blood shot or have spots in it. White is the color

	associated with Lung and Metal in the Five Element chart.
Pupil	Kidney and Water Water is the element of Kidney and is associated with the color black on the Five Element chart.
Iris	Liver and Wind Wood is associated with both Liver and Wind and also with the color green – in the digital book I was able to use color and the model's eye was green. Sorry. IDK, color it in with marker?

A couple of examples of using this theory for diagnosis:
- A patient with Spleen deficiency issues and damp retention might have swollen or puffy eyelids.
- If the entire eye is red, swollen, and painful this can indicate external wind and heat, or it can be related to Liver Fire rising up
- A worried and anxious patient will generate Ht fire and then their inner and outer canthus will get redder.
- Dark area around the eye on the skin can indicate a Kidney deficiency or damp and cold retention.

Other things you should note when observing the eye:
- Luster to the eyes
- Ability of patient to control eye movement
- Color of the eyes
- Bulging of the eyes can indicate hyperthyroidism, goiter, Liver Qi stagnation with phlegm retention. Bulging of one eye could be a tumor – Refer! Refer! Refer!

OBSERVATION OF THE NOSE

The nose is related to the following organs:

Organ	Connection to the Nose
Stomach	Connects to the nose through a branch of the Stomach channel that flows through the face.
Du	Du channel goes right down the center of the face and through the nose.
Bladder	Bladder channel goes to the bridge of the nose.
Large Intestine	Both the main and musculotendinous channel go to the bottom of the nose.

In the event you haven't heard about them yet, there are a bunch of microsystems around the body. Microsystems are reflections of the whole body in one part of the body. You will learn about 2nd metacarpal bone therapy and auriculotherapy later on in your advanced acupuncture techniques studies. You can needle these microsystems to affect change in the whole body. You can also use these microsystems to diagnose problems in the body. Generally you do this with palpation, but you can also do it via observation.

The same is true for the nose. You don't needle it that often (except for a couple of select points *around* the nose) because there are so many nerve endings on the nose and it would hurt like hell. BUT, you can observe the nose and the area around the nose as part of your diagnosing process.

Here is how the nose relates to the internal organs.

Organ/channel	Part of the nose that connects to
Lung	Area above the nose, between the eyebrows
Heart	Area between the inner canthi
Liver	Bridge of the nose
Gallbladder	Sides of the bridge of the nose
Spleen	Tip of the nose
Stomach	Sides of the nose
Bladder	Philtrum – top lip to the bottom of the nose Bladder itself, urinary tract, urogenital area in general

So what are you looking for here?

Looking for	Examples
Red coloration	Red = heat. Pretty much always, anywhere. A red, swollen nose can = damp + heat in St, Sp, Lv. Pretty common to see in alcoholics.
Swelling	Swelling = dampness.
Greasy nose	Damp and phlegm.
Flaring nostrils	Also called "flapping alae nasa." Nostrils flare with every inhale. Common to see in asthmatics
Nose bleeds	Ask how long it's been happening. Is it acute/excess or chronic/deficient? What color is the blood? Bright red indicates excess, dark/pale/watery indicates deficiency
Polyps	Lots of interpretations for all of these, but nothing that's likely to show up on a test. If you are really into this, there are whole schools of diagnosis based on nose observation. I'd encourage you to start reading!
Ulcers	
Frequent pimples	
Papules	

Let's just take a minute to be real, shall we?

Are you going to use every single one of these methods each time you walk into the clinic room to treat someone? No. Not unless you have about 3 hours to do an intake on each patient, which you don't!

But it could very well be that you walk in, say hello to your patient, and notice right away that this guy has a swollen, red nose and an ulcer on his mouth. If you're familiar with your diagnostics, you're going to make a quick note of it, realize that red always = heat, and then take a hot second after your full interview to go back and take a look at these notes.

Observation of Philtrum, Lips and Mouth, Teeth and Gums

Philtrum

The philtrum is the vertical divot you have between the top of the upper lip and the bottom of the nose. This area reflects the health of the Urinary Bladder, the urinary tract, and the urogenital area. The lower part of the philtrum also reflects the health of the uterus.

Does the patient have a burning pain when he or she urinates, for example? The color and quality you see in the philtrum can tell you what's causing it. If it looks redder than the surrounding tissue, for instance, it's probably heat.

Lips and Mouth

Dry lips, as an example, can reflect Body Fluid deficiency. Very red lips could indicate heat.

But the big takeaway, and you know that because I'm putting it in bold, is **drooping lips reflect Spleen Qi deficiency**.

Teeth and Gums

Teeth are considered to be a surplus of bone and are therefore related to Kidney. Kidney deficiency will manifest as problems with the teeth – loose teeth, teeth that break easily, easily get cavities, have a lot of plaque problems, color is weird, etc.

Channels that influence teeth and gums:

Channel	Area of influence
Stomach	Upper gums. Red upper gums = St heat
Large Intestine	Lower gums. Red lower gums can indicate heat in the LI, maybe constipation
Kidney	Both teeth and gums. Receding gums can = Ki deficiency
Du	Affects both teeth and gums.

Here are some common gum problems and how you could interpret them.

Problem	Possible interpretation
Gum inflammation	Full/excess or empty/Yin xu* heat in the St or LI
Bleeding gums	Sp Qi xu* so it cannot hold the blood in the vessels. Could also be empty heat due to St or Ki deficient fire.
Bleed, red, swollen gums	Now you're adding heat to the mix, so you are looking at heat or fire in the Stomach or LI.
Receding gums	Depending on the presentation, this could be Qi and Blood xu, St fire, or Ki yin xu with empty heat.
Gums oozing pus (acute)	St fire
Gums oozing pus (chronic)	Severe deficiency of Qi and Blood (probably leading to stagnation and then to heat).
Pale gums	Deficiency or cold
Red gums	Heat, either excess or deficient
Purple gums	Stasis condition

*Xu = deficiency in Chinese/Pinyin

OBSERVATION OF THE EARS

The ears are another of the many microsystems around the body. Auricular acupuncture is also a great way to treat the whole body, but observation of the ears can also tell you an awful lot about the condition of the body.

Several channels enter and influence the ears, either through the main channel or through a secondary or connecting channel.

Gallbladder – main channel	San Jiao – main channel
Small Intestine – main channel	Bladder – main channel
Stomach – main channel	Liver – connecting and collateral channels

Again, there are whole studies about just the ears. A French doctor in the 1950's, Paul Nogier, discovered that the ear connects to every part of the body and can be used to treat every part of the body. I'm not going to get into too much detail about ears and what each of these things mean here, but there are a couple of things you should note for now.

The size of the ears are probably the most clinically significant thing to know now.

Size of the Ears	Interpretation/s
Large ears	These are considered to be good luck, good health, good congenital Essence, and good Kidney Essence. Long earlobes are considered to be good fortune and long life. That's why so many Buddha images have huge earlobes. ….And what does that mean for people that put in the ear plug piercings? Hmmm.
Small ears or contracted ears	These are not so good. They reflect an Essence deficiency.

Without getting into too much interpretation, there are other things you might notice about the ears. Again, there are lots of studies and ear maps you could use to get a bead on what's happening in the body as it is reflected in the ears.

Problems	Possible interpretation/s
Swollen ears	Can reflect dampness in the body.
Dry and contracted helix	Yin xu, Fluid deficiency, other types of deficiency, depending on location on helix.
Sores	Note where they are and compare to auricular charts for location and interpretation. For colorations, refer to complexion charts and remember red = heat!
Warts on ears	
Abnormal coloration	
Distended blood vessels	
Excess ear wax production	Phlegm damp retention, infection or trauma to ear
Discharge	

Observations of the Nails

Nail surface abnormalities are related to Liver, Blood, and deficiency. Nails will change in both color and texture with deficiencies.

Problem	Possible interpretation
Ridges and indentations	Liver Blood xu or Liver Yin xu
White spots	Qi deficiency
Pale white color	Blood xu – Lv and Sp
Dull white color	Yang xu – Sp and Ki
Red	Generally a full heat
Yellow	Damp heat – St, Sp, Lv, Gb
Bluish color	Blood xu with internal cold
Greenish color	Severe Sp Qi xu + wind

Blue/green color	Blood stasis
Dark color	Ki yin xu, Ki yang xu, or Blood stasis
Purple or red/purple	Lv Blood stasis
Febrile disease + red/purple	Heat in the Blood

The lunulae of each of the the nails also has its' own significance.

Finger of lunulae	Correspondence
Thumb	Lung
Index finger	Heart
Middle finger	Spleen
Ring finger	Liver
Little finger	Kidney

OBSERVATIONS OF CHEST/ABDOMEN

Short and simple:

Presentation	Possible interpretation
Protruding chest	Chronic retention of phlegm, Liver Qi stagnation. Cat note: I've also known some chronic asthmatics who had this problem. Most likely phlegm retention.
Sunken chest	Lung Qi xu, Yin xu, Kidney xu. Cat note: I know a Marfan's Syndrome patient who has this sunken chest presentation too. Common in this patient population

OBSERVATION OF THE FOUR LIMBS

Also short and simple.

The Spleen relates to the four limbs. If the Spleen Qi is weak, the limbs will be also. And If the Spleen Qi is weak, then there's a good chance there is damp or Qi retention, which you can detect by checking for edema.

Type of Edema	Interpretation
Pitting edema (damp edema)	When you press on the front of the tibia, the impression stays for more than 120 seconds. Deficiency related. Likely to be Sp Qi xu and/or Ki Yang xu + dampness.
Non-pitting edema (Qi edema)	Definitely swelling, but when you press on the tibia, ankle, or top of foot the impression doesn't stay. Excess related. Likely to be a Qi stagnation and thus a Qi edema.

OBSERVATION OF BODY SECRETIONS

Really? People are going to show you their secretions? Admittedly, this isn't likely unless you are lucky enough to work in a hospital setting. But patients will talk about it with you. Bear in mind that sometimes they don't have the best perspective on the amount or the quality or the smell because people in a western population don't want to think about, much less talk about their excretions. This is why we invented toilet paper, tissues for blowing the nose, tampons, and flushing toilets!

With that in mind, I offer you this information.

The key points: you want to know the **amount of excretions, the color, the texture or property, and the smell**. See? It's in red, so it's important.

Smell? Yes, smell. Docs in the US largely don't do this any longer, I have witnessed other western trained doctors in other countries doing this routinely – they check for the smell of bodily excretions and of wounds that are healing.

Some examples about this:
- Damp phlegm retention might present as sputum that is large in volume, is white, loose, and has no smell.

- Urine that is deep yellow in color, scanty in volume, and has a strong smell is a problem of heat.
- Menstrual blood or vaginal discharge that is….
    - Pale colored, large volume, no or low smell can = a deficiency, probably of Qi.
    - Deep in color, has a strong smell, less volume is likely to be damp heat
    - Menstrual blood that is dark in color, has large clots is probably a Liver Qi stagnation

OBSERVATION OF THE SKIN

The big takeaways about skin: **red is heat, bright is fullness or excess, pale red is deficiency or emptiness**.

Presentation	Interpretation
Carbuncles	Collections of boils all clustered together in one painful hellacious area. These are swollen, red, large and painful, and often feel hot to the touch. This is heat, usually toxic heat, a Yang excess.
Furuncle	Another way to say boil. These are shallow, superficial, smaller than a carbuncle, and round. Usually aren't so red and swollen as a carbuncle. Sometimes transform into pus. Damp heat.
Nail-like boil	These are very small boils, but hurt nonetheless. The start the size of a grain of millet in the center, then slowly change until the root is very tight with white pus on top Toxic fire.

Gangrene	Woah! Jump from boils to gangrene! Yup. We did. Gangrene is the death of tissue caused by a truncated blood flow. Not pretty. The color of the skin will be dark and may be dry gangrene or wet gangrene. This is a Yin problem, usually Yin deficiency.

And of course, we have already talked about how color manifests on the skin, how dryness can present as dry skin, how sometimes Blood xu can present as dry rough skin, and so forth. So take all that into consideration when looking at a patient's skin too.

OBSERVATION OF THE ABDOMEN

Also short and sweet. There is a whole school of diagnosis involving palpation of the abdomen and what that means. Save it for later on when Chinese medicine is starting to make more sense to you. It's good stuff and well worth learning it later on though.

Here's what you want to know right now.

Presentation	Interpretation
Acute epigastric distention (often called focal distention)	Food stagnation in the Stomach
Epigastric and lower abdominal distention	Liver Qi stagnation
Distention of the abdomen + bowel disorder (like IBS, colitis, etc)	Qi stagnation in the intestines
Slight, chronic distention in the ab	Spleen xu
Severe distention of the abdomen	Damp phlegm retention

OBSERVATION OF CHILDREN

There **will** be test questions on this, probably both in your regular tests during your school career and later on the national boards. Personally, I always wanted to know more about treating kids, but my school didn't focus on it much, so we didn't get a ton about it. Later on I found a great text called *A Handbook of TCM Pediatrics*. If you're interested in treating children, check it out.

Here's what you need to now for now:

- This applies to kids less than 3 years of age. Once a kid gets older than that, they are developed enough that their bodies change and this no longer applies.

- The **index finger is the most important component in diagnosing children**. Pulses are too tightly packed for adult fingers to interpret them correctly, though I have seen a very talented pediatric acupuncturist lay her thumb across the whole pulse area to feel for wiry and slippery qualities. You can't really interview kids either – parents can give you some information, but they can't give you the subjective stuff at this age.

What you are looking for on kids is the superficial venule, indicated on the illustration by the black line. This vein runs up the medial side of the index finger and can give you some great clues as to what's happening in the child.

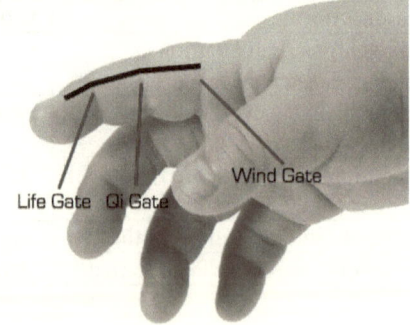

To diagnose this way, hold the child's wrist with your non-dominant hand, then lightly push this vein several times *from the tip of the finger*

toward the palm with your dominant hand. This squeezes the blood out of this vein so you can watch as it refills.

You are looking for both the *color* expressed in this vessel and *how far the color refills*. There are three segments to this vein you need to know. See the illustration above for the Gates in question below.

The Gate	Description and indication of disease severity
Wind Gate Feng Guan	Intersection of the vein and the 1st knuckle where the palm meets the finger joint at the crease. If the vein refills only to here, the prognosis is good and the disease is less severe.
Qi Gate Qi Guan	Intersection of the vein and the middle finger joint crease. If the vein refills to here, the prognosis is less awesome, the disease is more advanced, deeper in the body.
Life Gate Mind Guan	Intersection of the vein and the distal finger joint crease. If the vein refills this far, the prognosis is bad and the disease is severe, even life threatening.

Now let's talk about the colors you will see in this vessel when it is normal and when there is a disease condition.

Color	Indication
Slightly red, maybe a little bit yellowish	This is normal. No detectable disease present. The coloration will be faintly visible at the Wind Gate.
Purple/red	Interior heat syndrome This is a different color indication than it is in adults!

Purple and dark/black or blue/purple/black	Obstruction of blood vessels by phlegm, food, or heat. Indicates a severe problem.
Bright red vein	Exterior pathogens present. Also a different color presentation than you would see in an adult patient.
Blue/green	Convulsions, pain syndrome, or irregular food intake.
Quality of color	**Indication**
Color is light and fine	Deficiency of Qi and Blood
Color is deep, rough	Food retention in stomach and intestine

CHAPTER 6
Tongue Diagnosis

And now the moment you've all been waiting for: the moment you start looking at everyone's tongue all the time and can't stop.

I would consider the tongue to be yet another form of diagnostic microsystem. You can't really needle it – who would put up with that?! – but you can get an awful lot of information by looking at the tongue. As a matter of fact, you use pulse and tongue diagnosis to confirm what your other methods of observation, listening and smelling, questioning and such have revealed to you. If the pulse and tongue don't agree with what you're thinking, your clinic supervisor is going to argue with you about whether or not you're on the right track.

PREPARATION
Preparation? I gotta prepare for this? You do.

Lighting
You probably know that different types of light sources have different coloring. An incandescent bulb gives off a yellowish color. Flourescent and many of the LED bulbs have a bluish cast. Neither of these will reflect what's really happening with the tongue.

In the best case scenario, you look at a person's tongue in daylight using outdoor lighting, but standing in shade. If your clinic space has a window that gets good sunlight but you can be in a space where the sun *isn't* shining directly onto your patient's tongue, this is great.

If you are stuck in a totally indoor space or if opening your window would breach HIPPA in some way, using daylight spectrum bulbs in your lamps is the way to go.

Medications

Some medications can change the coloring of the tongue and the coating. Be sure to find out what medications a patient is on so that you can look it up and know how this will change the tongue color or remove the tongue coating. You don't want to go diagnosing someone with a Yin deficiency because you don't see a tongue coating when really they are just on a medication.

Foods and Drinks

I always ask my patients not to eat foods or drink things that will color their tongues before they come in for a treatment. Someone came to see me who had consumed a grape soda some hours earlier and her tongue was still purplish. It looked like a Blood stasis tongue, but then I found out about the soda. Blueberries, blackberries, popsicles, sodas, coffee, and a whole host of other foods and beverages will color the tongue body or coating. Always ask before you assume.

Tongue scraping

Tongue scraping has long been a practice in India and is now more and more common in the West. If you see a very thin coating or lack of coating, ask about this. Politely ask your patient not to scrape their tongue on the day of their next visit.

HOW TO LOOK AT THE TONGUE

Have your patient stick their tongue out

I need instructions for this? Yeah, you do. How far do they put their tongue out? For how long? What do you look at first? See? You need instructions.

How far to stick that thing out

Not so far that the patient has to strain to hold it out, but far enough that you can see all the way to the "root" of the tongue. Tongue should be soft and relaxed.

How long to keep it stuck out

No more than about 10-20 seconds. First, it gets tiring, the patient's tongue will start to feel cold and dry, it will actually start to look darker and drier as it's kept out longer, and you will notice more movement in the tongue. If you need more time to gaze longingly at the tongue, have them retract their tongue, shut their mouth, rest their tongue for about 10 seconds, then have them stick it back out and look a little more.

You can repeat this a couple of times in a row if you need to. After that the patient has about had it with that noise.

The tongue map

Look at the image here and notice how the tongue can function as a map to the internal organs. Pay attention to where you see the tongue body colors, tongue coatings, and any anomalies on the tongue.

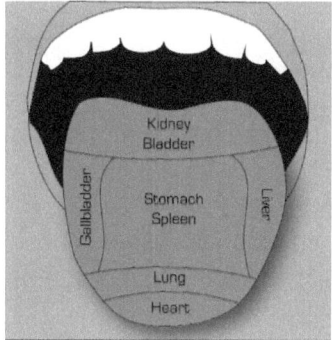

Diagnostics of Chinese Medicine: The Four Diagnostic Skills

The location of these things can give you an indication as to what is happening inside. For instance, if you see purple spots in the Liver area, you would take this as a possible clue of Liver Blood stasis. If you see a lack of tongue coating in the center area where it says Stomach/Spleen, you might be looking at a Stomach Yin deficiency. If the tip is very red, then possibly Heart fire.

Normal Tongue Presentation

You need to know what "normal" is before you can see what abnormal looks like.

Normal	More info
Color	Light red with brightness, or a 'shiny luster.' *
Movement	Soft and flexible
Body Fluid	Should be normal
Coating	Should be thin and white. Thin would be like a very sheer fabric over the light red coloring.
Veins under tongue	Light purple, not curved or "wiggly"

*My teacher had a thing about "luster." Dictionary.com says it means "a gentle sheen or soft glow" while Miriam-Webster says "a glow of light from within" and "a superficial attractiveness or appearance of excellence." So there you go. Pretty subjective. Does it have an appearance of excellence? Well, then it's normal!

Pathological Tongue Body Presentation

Color, shape, movement, and prickles on the tongue, can tell you about the health of the body.

Tongue body colors

I'm using 'xu' instead of deficiency to save space. Also, get used to seeing that. Common in a lot of writings and in chart notes, especially if you are reading chart notes from a Chinese colleague or instructor.

Body Color	Interpretation/s
Pale	Similar indications to pale face. • Qi xu – tongue might be more watery on surface • Yang xu – look for more cold signs to prove this – a yang xu is Qi xu + cold. • Blood xu – will have a drier appearance • Cold
Red	Red always indicates heat. Could be excess or xu. • Xu heat – thinner body, possible cracks on the surface as Yin xu continues. If severe, dark red in color (often called "scarlet" in writings). Might have very little coating, areas of missing coating (called "mapped"), or no coating at all ("mirror coating"). Mirror coating is common if you see St Qi xu + Yin xu. . . or when your patient has scraped their tongue! • Excess heat – bright red in color as opposed to light red normal tongue. • A patient's tongue will be redder if they have just eaten. Foods can also affect tongue body and coating color.
Deep red	This is the 'scarlet' coloring mentioned above in Xu heat.

Purple	• Blood stasis. Could be all over, or in spots
	   o Purple + moist = cold → stasis
	   o Purple + dry = Blood heat → stasis
	
	Dark distended vessels under tongue also signal Blood stasis

Tongue body shape and other anomalies

Shape	Interpretation/s
Thin	This is thin from side to side – kind of like a bird. Yin xu. Can be accompanied by thirst, hot flashes, night sweats, palm heat and/or all the other Yin xu s/sx.
Swollen	• Spleen Qi xu + damp retention. Will likely have teeth marks too. See that section of this table for more. • Yang excess (aka full/excessive heat). Will also appear red
Teeth marks	This is edema on the tongue, which causes the tongue to press against the teeth giving the tongue a kind of scalloped edge. Signals damp retention and probably Spleen Qi xu also.

Cracks or fissures	Similar to earth that has been sunbaked way too long.
	
	• Yin xu
	  May also present with little to no coating
	  ○ Ht Yin xu = Heart crack down the midline from tip back to Kidney
	  ○ Dryness + Yin xu
	• Blood xu + heat
	• Excess/full heat
	  Burns Yin and Body Fluids, causing cracking
	
	May also be totally normal if the patient has had this since childhood.

Prickles	These are red dots on the tongue you can see through the coating. They look kind of like measles. These indicate a heat condition. Pay attention to where the prickles are to give you an idea where the heat is. Prickles on the tip, for example could indicate heart heat.
Deviation	Wind Stroke - tongue pulls to left or to right side.

Tongue body movement

If your patient is unable to comfortably keep their tongue still either there is a pathology to this or you've simply had them keep their tongues hanging out too long.

Movement	Interpretation/s
Tremors	Think Liver Wind.
Quivering	Less severe than a full tremor. Can be due to Sp Qi and/or Blood xu.

PATHOLOGICAL TONGUE COATINGS

Coating presentations are only one component of tongue diagnosis and should be taken into consideration as part of the whole. I can only think of one instance in which the coating alone is a primary indicator (the tofu-like coating). This is why I'm presenting them as part of the whole tongue picture.

Some basic rules of thumb.
- A thin coating is one you can see through. It's somewhat transparent. Thin can indicate:
  o Normal coating
  o Exterior or superficial problem
  o Acute or early stage of a disease or syndrome
  o Very very thin can indicate a developing Yin xu.

- A thick coating is one you *can't* see through. You can't even tell what color the tongue body is through a thick coating. If you can't see the tongue body, look at the tip and sides for the body color.
    o Can indicate an interior or deeper problem
    o Longer lasting or chronic stage of disease
    o Excess of some kind
- Tongue coatings can change really quickly.

Tongue presentation	Interpretation/s
White coating	Can be normal
Yellow coating	Usually indicates heat
Grey coating	Indicates heat and/or damp cold. Often a sign that damp cold is turning into damp heat
Black tongue coatings	Black tongue coatings can be extreme heat or extreme cold. Look at the color of the tongue body and other s/sx to figure out which. Also, if someone takes charcoal tablets or other charcoal based supplements, this can turn the tongue coating black.
Thin white coating Body = pale, swollen	Spleen Qi xu with damp retention.
Thick white coating you can't see through Body=pale, swollen	Sp Qi xu with damp retention, but thicker coating you can't see through means condition has progressed and is much worse.
Yellowish coating Body=pale, swollen, teeth marks, reddish tip	Sp Qi xu with damp retention, but with heat (yellow). Reddish tip tells you the Ht is experiencing some heat too.
Yellow, thick, greasy, dry looking coat Body=red	- Yellow and red =heat - Thick = more severe, interior - Greasy/dry* = damaged body fluids This is internal heat.

Tofu-like coating	Also called "bean curd" coating. Thick coating you can't see through, but scapes off very easily. Will sometimes look yellow. You can see the margins of it on the edges of the tongue. Looks kind of rough and grainy. Indicates food stagnation/food retention or damp/phlegm. If yellow, there is some heat to the stagnation.
Greasy, thick coating	Smoother and finer with no graininess when compared to the bean curd coating, but looks kinda similar. Can't see the margins of this coating, can't scrape it off easily. Damp/phlegm retention.
Slippery	Similar to the greasy coating, but wetter and oilier. Damp/phlegm retention
Peeled or mapped coating	This is a Yin deficiency tongue. Pay attention to where the coating is missing. Gives you clues as to what organ/s is/are affected Looks like the coating has been exfoliated or peeled off in spots, so the coating resembles a geographical map.
Mirror coat	No coating at all. This is also a Yin deficiency tongue coating. Usually indicates a severe St Qi and Yin xu.

*Greasy tongue coatings + heat signs can indicate that heat has burned away some of the Body Fluids. Normal tongue coating is moist. This has a drier quality than that, but isn't totally dry yet. Greasy can also indicate phlegm, which also makes sense in the presence of heat cooking damp down into phlegm.

If the coating looks dry and greasy, that's heat damaging the Body Fluids. If it looks more moist and greasy, then you're looking at damp heat.

This page intentionally, whole-heartedly, and enthusiastically left blank.

SECTION 2:
LISTENING AND SMELLING

What can I say? The whole short section is about listening and smelling.

This page intentionally left blank.

CHAPTER 7
Listening

Listening is different than asking questions and doing a patient intake. This is listening to the sounds the body makes when it inhales and exhales, to the vocal quality, for abnormal languaging, and for digestive sounds. What do your ears tell you about this patient?

Before you ever start asking questions, notice this first. This is why some docs will make small talk with you. It's a form of evaluation. Does your voice sound ok? Are you coughing, sneezing ,wheezing, sniffling? How's your overall emotional tone? Do your sentences seem cohesive and make sense?

LISTENING TO THE VOICE

Not the words – the voice. What if you couldn't speak this person's language and heard them talking? What would you notice about their vocal sounds? What kind of noises does this human make with their vocal cords?

Sounds	Interpretation/s
Louds voice	Lung Qi is strong….or there is an excess Zhong qi is also related to this, but focus on the Lung.

Hoarse voice	To find out why, use all of your diagnostics skills
	Some examples:
	• Short term duration – could be…
	   o Wind cold or wind heat invasion
	   o Respiratory infection/common cold
	   o Speaking too much
	   o Dryness – maybe heat damaging Body Fluids

	• Long term, chronic in duration could be…
	    ○ Deficient heat drying body fluids
	    ○ Yin deficiency (most likely)
	    ○ Tumor or cancer due to Blood stasis

Children crying at night	This is abnormal crying, not a kid who just doesn't want to go to bed. • Food stagnation – causes heat to accumulate in the St and Sp and is uncomfortable. • Fright

ABNORMAL LANGUAGE

There is range of things that are considered abnormal speech in Chinese medicine which are indicative of interior problems.

Manifestation	Interpretation/s
Delirium	Speech that makes no logical sense. Delirium (as opposed to dementia) comes on very quickly. High fevers can cause this. It also happens to elderly patients, often as the first sign of a severe UTI or bladder infection.* • Heat disturbing the Shen • Heat entering the Pericardium.
Murmuring to one's self	Heart Qi deficiency is one reason for this.
Excessive talking, won't quiet down**	Heat and excesses will do this.
Won't talk at all	Deficiency and cold will sometimes manifest this way.

*Still can come down to internal heat disturbing the Shen, Heart, and/or Pericardium. Why? Because the Bladder channel – the foot *Taiyang* – is connected to the Small Intestine – the hand *Taiyang* – and the Small Intestine channel is connected to the Heart.

**Have the patient stick out their tongue to quiet them down. You can also treat them face down to help their mind and their heart settle down.

LISTENING TO RESPIRATION

Listen to the sound a person's breathing makes. If they have a respiratory infection or phelgm retention in the Lung, you can hear this when they breathe. You can hear the rattle in the chest, the tone of the voice, you can hear hoarseness. You can do this with just your ears or with your stethoscope. All of that counts!

Some notes on asthma.

Asthma has an acute and a chronic phase. The acute phase is characterized as an excess while the chronic or less severe phase is considered to be a deficiency. So an asthma patient has both!

The acute phase is often triggered by the environment. That can be dust, pollen, a sudden shift from heat to cold. During this phase you will see the patient struggling to breathe. They will often breathe through an open mouth, lift their shoulders on the inhale, and their nostrils will flare on the inhale as well. We look for something called The Three Depressions: 1) depression at the tracheal notch, and 2) the two areas right above the clavicles. You will see these areas get more "hollow" on the patient's inhales.

If you listen with a stethoscope you will likely hear wheezing, which is the air moving through and over phlegm in the respiratory system.

During the deficiency phase, the chronic phase, a patient may feel they can breathe normally, but you will detect low voice volumes and occasional shortness of breath even though there is no wheezing or coughing.

COUGHING

Coughing is likely to occur when the weather changes from warm to cold, or from dry to wet.

Sometimes patients will also report coughing related to posture changes, though they don't usually express it like that. For instance, patients will talk about coughing a lot when they wake up in the morning. Why is that? A lot of phlegm is generated at night but the patient is quiet and quiescent. When they sit up or stand up in the mornings, the Qi and therefore the phlegm starts moving and the Lung wants to clear it out. Hence the coughing.

The reverse of this happens at night. The Qi and the phlegm settles into whatever position you are in, so during the day it finds a 'place' in the Lung and sits still. Lying down at night shifts this balance, so the Qi and the phlegm move around again.

Always ask how long patients have had a cough, if there is phlegm and if so is it loose/sticky/white/clear/yellow, easy to cough up or not, dry or wet.

Some basic indications about cough:

Type of cough	Interpretation/s
Dry cough	Yin deficiency. Burns and dries the fluids, dryness will irritate the throat.
Wet cough	Phlegm and damp
Loud cough	Like a loud volume or a barking cough – indicates an excess and it's probably acute not chronic.
Soft cough	Deficiency

DIGESTIVE NOISES

You'll cover more about digestive noises in your biomedical studies classes – listening for bowel sounds and how to do that. For now, here's what you need to know from the Chinese medicine perspective:

Vomiting

Are you likely to hear someone vomiting in clinic? It happens, but not that often. But you can ask questions about it and people will often tell you. This stuff is also handy to know if you have kids. If you've never heard your kids vomit, then you are probably raising a robot army.

Vomiting is about the rebellion of Stomach Qi. The Stomach is supposed to descend food downward. When it can't the energy has to go somewhere and that's upward.

Vomit sounds	Interpretation/s
Loud, projectile	This is an excess. Verify that it is an acute condition. Betcha it is.
Low sound, chronic	Chronic condition of Stomach rebellion.

Hiccups

This is also a Stomach Qi rebellion. Qi should be descending, but the energy is moving upward through the vocal cords and making the noises. Ask how long it's been going on and listen for how loud the hiccups are.

Hiccup sounds	Interpretation/s
Long term, quiet sounds	Deficiency – either deficient cold or deficient heat affecting the Stomach
Short term, loud	Excess Stomach cold or excess Stomach heat If it's heat, use St 44 to clear the heat in the organ and channel

This page intentionally left blank

CHAPTER 8
Smelling

I was in Mexico and helped treat an elderly patient who had developed a bed sore. One day when I was in her hospice room her doctor came by. (Yes, docs in Mexico actually still do house calls.) He changed her dressing and I saw him smell the bandages. When I asked what he was doing he told me about how he and other doctors in Mexico routinely smell patients as part of their diagnostic process when they are looking for signs of infection. Though it is not common practice in the US medical community, smell has long been an important indicator of health. Here are some notes on it as it pertains to Chinese medicine.

BELCHING SMELLS

Everybody belches which is no problem unless it is very frequently (Stomach Qi isn't descending, food is sitting and outgassing) or it smells bad. Belching with a fetid odor can signal food stagnation or food retention.

More common in kids than in adults. Look at the tongue and check for the bean curd coating mentioned in the section on tongue diagnosis. Gas, bloating and perhaps diarrhea are also possible s/sx you might see with smelly belching. Check the pulse for a slippery, tight, or choppy feel.

ROTTEN APPLE SMELL

Rotten apple smells – appley, but sickly sweet – indicates diabetes. The smell comes from ketones that build up in the blood due to a high blood sugar count. You'll get way more on diabetes later, but for now, know that diabetes can be either Type 1 or Type 2.

Type 1 diabetes used to be very early onset and is generally due to a failure of the pancreas to produce sufficient insulin. Type 2 diabetes used to be adult onset diabetes that was due to chronic high blood sugar and/or pancreatic inability to keep up with insulin demand. In the past couple of decades however, after high fructose corn syrup become the norm, the incidence of Type 2 diabetes in children has been increasingly common.

As a rule, Type 1 Diabetes has been viewed as a yin deficiency. Patients are often slender, younger, and have a high thirst drive. Type 2 Diabetes, which is still more frequently seen in adults as compared to kids, is generally seen as a phlegm damp retention problem. Overweight patients will sometimes be diabetic and not even know it.

OTHER DISTURBING SMELLS

Smell	Interpretation/s
Fetid smelling phlegm	Often with pus and blood in the sputum. This is a Lung carbuncle or "fei yong" in Chinese. Think staphylococcus or even tuberculosis (though tuberculosis is less common in the US than it used to be).
Ammonia smells	Kidney deficiency of some kind
Halitosis	Strong breath smell. Generally indicative of some level of Stomach heat. • Excess heat: strong sense of hunger, bitter taste in the mouth, thirsty for cold drinks, doesn't like touch. • Deficient heat: chronic, dull pain in the stomach, feels better with touching, very little hunger, wants either warm or cool drinks and has low level thirst. •
Menstrual smells	• Strong smelling = excess or heat • Little or no smell = deficiency

Section 3:
Asking Questions

You'd think this would be part of Listening, right? Not so much. Listening refers to the *sense* of listening and taps the intuitive senses. Asking Questions and getting answers engages the language and interpretation centers of the brain.

There are several sets of questions that are standard in Chinese medicine. Know them well and, better yet, understand why they are asked!

Left blank for your non-reading pleasure.

CHAPTER 9
The Ten Traditional Questions

The minute you greet a patient the interview has begun. The first skill you use is always observation. You are watching and evaluating even when you first greet them. You talk with them a bit and you are using listening skills to hear the noises their body tends to make.

And then you get to the asking part. This is a very important information gathering tool and *can be* more straightforward than any of the others. . . so said my Chinese professors. I actually kind of disagree. I find that people forget their own history and cover stuff up they are embarrassed about, even when it would help you understand better and give them a better diagnosis and treatment.

Example:
I was watching one of my professors do a patient intake one afternoon. He asked the woman if she had any difficulty sleeping and she said no, never. He moved on. Later in the interview he asked if she was on any medications. Nope, never. But when he asked about over the counter meds she replied, "Oh! Yes! I take 2 Tylenol PMs every night."

And that explained why she never had any trouble going to sleep! But if he hadn't somewhat casually asked about over the counter meds, we might not have known that indeed, she had chronic insomnia but had been self medicating for it for the past several years.

After your intake, you will move on to the pulse and tongue analysis.

THE BASICS OF INTERVIEWING

1. Use all of your skills
   You must combine all of your skills together to get a clear and complete picture about what is happening with your patient.

2. Talkative vs. quiet patients
   Some people are normally more verbose than others. Never directly interrupt or be rude. You want people to trust you with information, which they will not if they find you brash or harsh. You must learn to guide and redirect talkative patients. Equally important, you have to learn how to draw information out of quiet folks.

   Talking skills are hard if you're an introvert like me who sucks at small talk. Time to learn new skills!

3. Patient confidentiality
   Conversations in the clinic are confidential. Learn your HIPPA laws and abide by them at all times. United States law is very clear about this – you can never mention patients' names or signs and symptoms. As a matter of fact, most practitioners won't even greet patients out in public for fear that this will be a breach of confidentiality. If the patient greets you first, then cool. They don't mind people knowing they are associated with you.

   Don't take the snub personally if they *don't* greet you. There are a myriad of reasons they might not want others to know they are getting acupuncture or seeing a practitioner. As an example, I know a woman whose husband has strong religious beliefs that acupuncture is a sin. But acupuncture is the only way she can manage her stress, so she just doesn't tell him about going to see an acupuncturist. Obviously, if her acu ran up to her to say hello in public, things could get awkward. Always let U.S. patients approach you first.

This is not necessarily true in other countries. Always find out about the laws in whatever country you practice in!

4. Ask about the chief complaint first.
   This is what your patient is coming to you for. Ask the heck out of this. This is why they are here – they want to be heard and they want to talk about this!

5. Keep an open mind.
   There were times in student clinic when I just *knew* I was right about something and it turns out I either wasn't or missed something really important because I'd already made a judgment. Don't do that.

   Also keep an open mind about what the patient is telling you and what the s/sx are. Or what their values are. Or whatever. We aren't in the clinic to judge people, but to help them at whatever level they are at.

   I once had a patient who I knew could shift her life by changing her diet, but she wasn't ready to hear that for a couple of years. Finally, 3 years after I started treating her, dropping hints about how dairy was probably producing more phlegm, was combining with heat, and making it impossible for her to sleep, she asked what she could do herself so she didn't have to come to acupuncture 3 times per week in order to sleep. I suggested some dietary substitutions and she was ready to hear it. She "fixed herself" with diet and didn't need acupuncture as often!

Don't judge a patient as non-compliant when they just aren't ready to make the bounce to something different.

GETTING A FULL HISTORY

The first time you see someone, if you haven't seen a patient in a long time, or if you see someone regularly, but it's been a couple of years since the last full intake, you need a full history. Here's what you need.

The Chief Complaint

Sometimes abbreviated CC on charts.

- *Always* start here. If the patient gives you a ton of information, you need to narrow it down to a cohesive, concise sentence. Many softwares and chart notes give you about 2 lines for the Chief Complaint. Word it short and simple.

- This should come from the patient, not the practitioner. This is not the time for a diagnosis, but for the patient's main reason for coming to see you. Here's a good example and a bad example.
    - Good CC: Headache for 2 weeks, worse last 24 hours.
      This gives the reason that motivated the patient to seek help, tells you how long it's been happening and that it has increased in intensity recently.

    - Bad CC: Hypertension for 1 year.
      Hypertension is a *diagnosis*, not a chief complaint. You also don't know if the 1 year thing is true or if the whole diagnosis is correct. This is an example of taking the report of another practitioner's diagnosis as fact when it might not be true. The

patient may have mis-reported, the diagnosis might be off.

A number of years ago one of my patients said she had been told by her doc that she had diabetes. None of the symptoms fit, yet her doctor was pressing her to begin taking metformin. I sent her to another western med doc for a 2nd opinion who did a thorough range of tests and she came up definitively negative for diabetes. Upon further investigation, we discovered it was a clerical error in the input of an ICD code. She'd *never* had diabetes.

Takeaway: Never assume that the diagnosis of another practitioner is correct. Make your own diagnosis based on CC and supporting data.

- A good chief complaint includes the length of time the patient has had the problem. This tells you if the problem is acute or chronic. That can drastically change how you treat the problem.

Present History

This is the history surrounding the Chief Complaint.

The things you want to know:

- How did the problem start? When and what started it?
- What have you tried to resolve it so far?
- What makes it better? What makes it worse?
- What are the signs and symptoms right now?

Past History

This is less related to the Chief Complaint possibly, but puts the CC into context in the life of this person. You will see tons of past history type questions on intake forms that go further than this.

- Other past diseases and health challenges
  Surgeries?
  Qi and Blood stagnation and stasis is the pathological product of past surgeries. Helps you make differentiations sometimes.

Personal History

Where the Past History goes into medical history, this is about lifestyle. Some examples:

- Appetite.
  What the patient likes to eat, craves most of the time, what are the eating habits, etc.

- Alcohol consumption
  Beer, or instance, tends to add to damp retention in the body. Even an answer like, "I used to drink, but stopped because I was getting leg cramps at night after drinking" can be incredibly useful.

- Smoking
  Smoke leads to lung deficiency and skin dryness among other things.

- Recreational drug use
  Most people won't disclose this at first. The drug laws in the United States are pretty draconian and the penalties are pretty awful, so a lot of people are reticent

to even disclose marijuana usage. Regular drug use can indicate addiction problems.

Family History

Great stuff to know since some things follow families. I was lucky enough to get to treat several whole families and got to see how mothers and children shared certain tendencies and s/sx. Liver Qi stagnation, though common in the U.S. population, can take very different forms. Not in one particular family! They shared the same expression in all of the kids and the mom.

Allergies, cancers, heart conditions, diabetes, even menstrual dysfunctions can fall along family lines. Cancer is almost always related to blood stasis, coronary heart disease to phlegm retention, etc.

THE TEN TRADITIONAL QUESTIONS

Though there are only 10, there are things to know about each... of course!

1. Aversion to chills, fever

When a patient reports chills and a fever, ask questions like:
- When did it start?
  Establishes
- Do you know what caused it?
  (Example: Walking home in the rain, woke with chills and a fever the following day.)
- Do you have more fever, less chills? Equal amounts? More chills, less fever?
  These answers will help you understand something important about what's happening. *Always verify with other s/sx!*

Chill/fever %	Interpretation/s
Chills and fever are =	That's the very **beginning of an exterior syndrome**.
Chills > Fever	Patient feels mostly cold, a little bit, low fever. When chills are greater than fever, this indicates a **wind cold invasion at the exterior** of the body.
Fever > chills	Indicates a **wind heat invasion on the exterior**.
Chills only	No fever, only chills. If it started as an exterior syndrome and progressed to chills only, this is now **interior cold**. • If excess, is probably somewhat acute and is not relieved by warming therapies (wrapping up, electric blankets, hot showers, etc.) • If deficient, will show yang deficiency s/sx and will feel better with warming therapies.
Fever only	No chills, just fever. Indicates interior heat syndrome. • Excess: high fever, plus interior heat s/sx. • Deficient: fever is lower than in excess condition, often varies during the day. Look for confirming Yin xu s/sx.
Alternating chills and fever	Don't have them at the same time, but they seem to alternate back and forth. This is **half exterior, half interior**. Six Channel Theory which you will get in the 2nd book of Diagnostics, details how contagious diseases progress from Taiyang → Yangming → Shaoyang →Taiyin, → Shaoyin → Jueyin stages. In the first 2 stages the disease is on the exterior. In the

	final 3 stages the disease is on the interior and getting deeper in the body. Shaoyang is the stage at which the disease is moving from exterior to the interior and is characterized by this alternating chills and fever.

2. Sweating

Here's what you ask about sweating and what that indicates.

Sweating Q's	Interpretation/s and discussion
When do you sweat?	Day, night? Moving or sitting? • During the day, sweat heavily during movement = Yang of Qi deficiency • At night or even during the day during a nap = Yin deficiency
Where do you sweat?	Sweating in a single area can tell you what organ might be affected. Sweating all over might indicate an exterior condition. There is something called exterior sweating and another something called interior sweating. More on that below.
Nature of the sweating?	• A cold sweat can indicate Yang xu • A hot sweat can indicate Yin xu

Exterior and interior sweating? What? That means sweating in the case of an exterior syndrome vs sweating in the case of interior syndromes. Let's break it down.

Exterior Sweating	Interpretation/s and discussion
Sweat + fast, superficial pulse	Exterior heat. Look for wind heat s/sx + red tongue body with a thin, yellow coating.
Little sweating + superficial/tight pulse	Exterior cold. Cold closes the pores. This is a kind of exterior excess, but not as excess as the

	last example in this table.
Sweating + slowed/lazy pulse	Exterior deficiency That's an exterior invasion of some kind plus the patient has a Wei Qi or Lung Qi type deficiency and can't sweat out whatever it is that's trying to invade. Could be a wind cold invasion that would normally slam the sweat pores shut, but the body is too weak to even slam the door.
Zero sweating + superficial and tight pulse	Exterior excess. Body is relatively strong and those sweating pores are slammed tightly shut.
Interior Sweating	**Interpretation/s and discussion**
General Sweating • Spontaneous sweating all over – day	Qi deficiency or Yang deficiency
• Spontaneous sweating all over – night	Yin deficiency
• Profuse sweating	If one of the 4 Bigs (high fever, big sweats/thirst/pulse), then Yangming stage of the Six Channels.
• Shivering + sweating	Called Zhan Han in Chinese (sweat shiver). • If pulse comes down and fever drops afterwards = good prognosis • If patient is restless, fast pulse, fever continues = bad prognosis
Local Sweating – only sweating in one area	
• Head only	Upper jiao, damp heat
• Palms/soles	Spleen/Stomach damp heat
• One side of the body only	Channel is blocked on the non-sweating side.

3. Head and Body

Questions to ask about the head and body. You'll notice everything in these charts are about pain. Also notice the different types of headaches as defined in TCM. You'll get a lot of questions about this over your learning and testing life and it comes up in clinic – like a *lot*.

Headache q's	Interpretation/s and discussion
When did you get the headache?	Establishes acute (recent acquisition – possibly excess) vs chronic (long term – deficiency)
Where is the headache? This is *extremely* significant. **KNOW these types and their locations.**	
• Forehead	Yangming headache The Foot Yangming (ST) meridian goes to the forehead.
• Vertex/top of head	Jueyin headache Very LV related, as that channel goes to the vertex.
• Occipital area	Taiyang headache The BL channel has points on the back of the neck and back of the head. Think tension headache from sitting and studying too much. "Texting neck" affects this area too.
• Temples	Shaoyang headache The GB channel (Foot Shaoyang) has points on the temples. Shaoyang headaches can also involve the LV meridian.
• Whole head	Shaoyin headache The KI channel goes deep into the head. This headache is probably chronic. Headaches that are behind the eyeball are also considered Shaoyin headaches.

	Qi and Blood deficiency, KI and LV Yin deficiency headaches tend to go throughout the whole head and often feel "empty." Note: Chronic headache pain inside the head can be a symptom of cancer, tumor.
What is the nature of the pain?	
• Throbbing/pulsing pain	LV Yang rising is the common cause. A full on LV fire can cause this type of pain too. Could also be a precursor to an aneurysm.
• Distending pain	LV Yang rising, also called Excessive LV Yang Similar to a balloon filling up in the head.
• Stabbing, fixed pain, worse at night	Blood Stasis related
• Dull pain	Often Qi and/or Blood deficiency + damp and phlegm retention.
• Heaviness + pain	Phlegm and damp – often happens in conjunction with a Yangming headache
• Penetrating pain	Cold causes this. Feels like the pain is penetrating into the body or head.
• Pain with empty feel	Qi and Blood deficiency, LV and KI Yin xu headaches. Pain is less severe and the head feels empty or hollow. See Whole Head headaches in the chart above.

Now on to body pain questions.

Body q's	Interpretation/s and discussion
Where is the pain?	Have them point and touch it. Way more reliable and faster than verbal descriptions or you palpating blindly around a general area.
How long have you had this pain?	Short time = excess/acute. Long time = chronic/deficiency.
What is the nature of the pain?	
• Sharp	Indicates an excess of some kind
• Dull	Deficiency, usually of Qi and Blood
• Fixed	Often is Blood stasis, especially if it is also like pins and needles, could be worse at night.
• Moving	Often a Qi congestion/stagnation
• Cold or hot in nature?	Tells you if it's aggravated by heat or cold. Also ask what makes it feel better – warm or cool? Gives you similar info.
• When does it occur?	Pain complaints are sometimes of a "comes and goes" nature. Stomach pain, for instance, may occur before eating which could indicate a stomach ulcer. Pain during eating is Stomach related, pain after eating is often Spleen/intestinal related, like a duodenal ulcer.
• Does it feel better or worse with touch or pressure?	Better with pressure = deficiency Worse with pressure = excess

4. Urine and Stool

While you aren't likely to *see* urine or stool all that often, you can always ask about it. If someone is new to acupuncture and alternative medicines they may have rarely if ever looked at their excrement. Or they may secretly look at it and not talk about it. Either way, you have to do a little bit of work to train your patients to notice and talk about this.

Like the naturalists and body archaeologists that we are, we learn a ton about people based on what their body discards and how.

Urine q's	Interpretation/s and discussion
What color is your urine? Normal urine is straw-colored – light yellow and without cloudiness.	
• Pale	Pale urine is indicative of cold and/or deficiency. KD xu, for instance, can result in pale, profuse urine.
• Dark yellow	The shade will vary, but darker yellows indicate heat. The more heat there is, the darker the yellow.
• Bright yellow	Jaundice.
• Reddened	Blood in the urine. Will look either red or orangey. Possibly due to excess heat in the Lower Jiao. Could be Sp Qi xu sufficient that Sp cannot hold the blood in the vessels. Could be bladder or kidney stones, will have back pain with kidney stones. Urination will sometimes stop spontaneously as stones more down the ureter. Hurts like bloody hell too.

How much urine do you produce? (Depends on liquid intake, obvs.)	
• Profuse	Excessive amounts that don't seem to match intake can be the result of a deficiency. Kidney Yang xu, for instance will cause profuse and very clear urine.
• Scanty	Indicates an excess in most cases, but can also be dehydration (poor fluid intake), Body Fluid deficiency, heat (xu or excess) burning off fluids.
How often do you go?	
• Normal	Depends on water and fluid intake. Rule of thumbs for this vary. If you pee every hour or two, you're probably good on water intake.
• Frequently	• Excess heat = frequent, urgent, burning, painful urine. Often darker yellow in color. • Deficient cold = profuse, clear color, incontinence Caffeine, soda, sugar intake can increase frequency. Caffeine increases the urge. Sugar is hard for the kidney to process due to the size of the molecules, which requires more water to push through the filters. So more urination.
Pain during urination?	Pain during urination is not normal. This is called Lin Syndrome. There are several types you will learn way more about later on in some of your treatment of disease classes. Some types due to Qi stagnation, Bloody Lin comes with blood and pain upon urination, there's a Heat Lin syndrome, Lin due to stones, and another due to STDs.

Stool Questions	Interpretation/s and discussion
What color is your poop? Ok, maybe don't say poop. Stool sounds more clinical.	
• Normal	Brown in color, not too light, not too dark.
• Pale or white stool	Lv/Gb Qi stagnation. Indicates the gallbladder isn't secreting bile. That's what gives poop the brown color. Stones or sludge can form in the Gb when the Qi isn't moving, blocks secretion of bile.
• Red in color or streaks of red	Indicates blood in the stool. *So* may reasons for this. The color indicates the blood hasn't been in the intestinal tract long, so it's a problem in the lower intestine such as a hemorrhoid, fissure, or intestinal ulceration. Often an indication of heat in the intestines or of hemorrhoids.
• Black or dark in color	Indicates blood in the stool but coming from higher up in the digestive tract. The longer the blood has been in the tract the more oxygen it loses and the darker it gets. The higher it is the tract, the blacker it will be. Likely a stomach or duodenal ulcer.
How frequently do you go?	
• 3+ times per day	This is diarrhea. Diarrhea is associated with loose or liquid stool, but really it's about frequency. If also watery, Sp Qi is not holding the liquids for processing. If more dysentery (smelly, maybe with blood or pus, painful) then probably damp heat – look for other confirming s/sx. If diarrhea every morning around 5am, probably Yang xu. The channels have different times per day! Check out the bio clock below. Pay attention to when diarrhea (and other sx) happen – can indicate what organ is affected.

• 3+ days since last bowel movement	Constipation is defined as more than 3 days without a bowel movement. How hard it is to get it moving is a different thing, but that's how any define it – hard to push out.

Can indicate Qi xu – not enough Qi to push the stool out, so sits in the bowels.
Can indicate heat damaging Body Fluids. You need fluid to lubricate the stool or it won't move. In Chinese this is referred to as 'not enough water to float the boat.' I kind of love that! |
| Formed or unformed? | Formed is considered normal – should show the shape of the intestines and hold together well.

Unformed is loose or watery or like a pile of sand or pieces that don't stick together. That indicates water retention and/or Qi stagnation.

The more like pebbles the stool is, the more dryness or heat is affecting the intestines. |
What is the odor like?	Very strong odors and smelly stool indicate heat and excess. No odor indicates deficiency and/or cold. Should be somewhere in between.
Is there any mucus present?	Indicates damp or phlegm retention.
Any burning sensations?	Burning usually indicates hemorrhoids, can be heat in the lower intestines.
If there is a problem with the stool, when did it start?	As with all of the when did it start questions, you're looking for acute (often excess) vs chronic (deficiency).

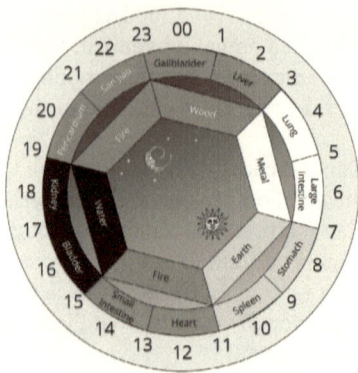

5. Eating and Drinking

Really, this should be drinking and eating because thirst questions tell you a tremendous amount and may be the more important question.

Drink questions	Interpretation/s and discussion
Do you get thirsty on a regular basis?	
• No	Might not be a bad thing. No might mean you have a patient that knows how to hydrate their body properly. (This hasn't been my clinical experience most of the time, but could happen! LOL.) No could also indicate a fluid metabolism problem like damp retention.
• Yes	"Yes" could be a good thing, indicating a normal thirst drive, but frequent thirst can also indicate a problem. If they have accompanying heat signs (red tongue with yellow coating, fast pulse, etc.) then thirst is a problem. Excessive thirst drive can also indicate a fluid metabolism problem in that the fluids aren't being distributed well.

Do you prefer hot or cold beverages?		
• Preference for warm/hot	Indicates cold internally	
• Preference for cold/cool	Indicates some level of internal heat.	
How much do you drink?		
• Large quantities	Can indicate excess heat, loss of fluids (diarrhea, vomiting, sweating, etc.), or a chronic problem hurting Ki Yin causing Yin xu heat.	
• Not a lot	Thirst without a desire to drink indicates 3 main things: • Yin xu heat Get confirming s/sx for this. Yin xu heat often leads to dry mouth and throat, so patient doesn't really want to drink, but wants to sip small amounts to moisten the mouth and throat. • Damp and/or phlegm retention with or without heat. Water distribution problem – there's enough of it, but it's not getting to the right places in the body. Example: phlegm damp retention in the St can cause nausea when patient drinks water. • Blood stasis. Doesn't really want to drink – has dry mouth and sip water or drink small amounts to moisten the mouth and throat. Might also have a purple tongue and other Blood stasis s/sx.	

Food questions	Interpretation/s and discussion
Do you crave anything on a regular basis? Cravings tell you what the body is looking for. This isn't a fleeting craving, but "I want this on a regular basis."	
• Spicy	Might be some kind of internal cold – excess or deficiency. Frequent indulgences in spicy foods can damage Yin.
• Sweet	Sp deficiency. Five element association of Earth is sweet. Frequent sweet eating can cause dampness
• Sour	Like pickles, lemon, etc. This is a symptom of Lv Qi stagnation.
• Salty	Kidney deficiency
How is your appetite?	
• Poor	Poor appetites can indicate may things. Often Sp xu, but can be St damp retention, and so much more. Examples: • Poor appetite with no tolerance for fried or oily foods + mild fever, yellowed skin and eyes = hepatits and jaundice with Lv and Gb damp heat • Poor appetite with belching and sour regurgitation + bean curd tongue = food retention. • Zero appetite + no menses and slippery pulses = morning sickness
• Good	Good appetites can be normal. Some dysfunctions don't impact the appetite at all. You can have good appetite, but then loose stool immediately after, which = St/Sp disharmony – strong St, weak Sp.
• Strong	Strong doesn't mean "good." Strong in this case is *too* strong. Strong + frequent is the implication here. Examples of dysfunctions: • Stomach fire = excessive almost constant hunger, usually with bad breath and pulse/tongue supporting this. • Hungry with no desire to actually eat = St deficient fire (from St Yin xu).

6. Chest and Abdomen Questions

Honestly? These are similar to the questions you asked in the Head and Body section and these are mostly about pain sensations also. I always want to know:

Where is the pain?
When did it start?
What is the nature of the pain?
What have you tried to make it better?
Is it better or worse if you touch it or press on it?
Is it better with warmth or cold?

And so forth.

Chest pain can be due to Qi stagnation in the chest, to a Lung Qi problem, or to a coronary or circulatory problem. In your biomedical classes you will learn a lot about heart problems, so we're going to leave that one for now.

Abdominal pain things you should note:

- Heart pain can refer to the stomach! Stomach pain may be a heart problem is what I'm saying.

- Abdominal pain that is acute and severe, may have fever, possible burning pain in which the abdomen feels rigid to the touch and worse with pressing indicate an excess, possibly a perforated ulcer. Patient may have a history of blackened stool.

- Abdominal pain could also be gallbladder related. Might have stones or sludge. Look for a colicky pain and a fever. Acupuncture can stop the pain temporarily, but these people need a referral to an ER.

- Pain starting in the stomach and moving to the lower right abdomen can be appendicitis. Abdomen may feel hard to the touch. You'll learn more about this in biomedical studies.

- Excessive diarrhea + abdominal pain that is too high to be intestinal can indicate pancreatitis.

7. Hearing and deafness

This question is often referred to just as Deafness, but includes varying levels of hearing problems and also tinnitus. This category is geared toward hearing difficulty and ringing in the ears. The basic questions are:

Do you have any difficulty hearing?
Do you have ringing in your ears?

You could go on with more questioning though. When I ask about ears and hearing, I generally want to know (if the answers indicate that there is a hearing related problem of some kind):

How long have you had the problem, what happened that might have caused it, did it come on suddenly or slowly (acute/excess or chronic/deficient), has there been any discharge (could indicate an infection), do you produce a lot of earwax (can indicate damp or phlegm), what have you tried, what seems to help, any pain, family history of this, etc.

A lot of these are similar to what you'd ask about anything going on in the body.

Hearing related information

A *bunch* of meridians cross the hearing centers in a very small space. Qi and Blood tend to flow slowly through this area. Honestly, deafness is difficult to treat and success varies. The more acute the deafness, the harder it seems to be to treat it.

True deafness is a total blockage and is an excess. Someone who cannot hear clearly, who isn't totally deaf, could be suffering from Lv Wind, Lv Heat, Ki deficiency, Yin xu affecting the Lower Jiao (causing Yang to float upwards), and more.

Hearing difficulties can also be medication related.

Tinnitus

Tinnitus is a ringing, buzzing, or other sounds in the ears that patients can hear intermittently, frequently, or constantly. It can be due to malnourishment or even partial blockage.

Some tinnitus points to ponder:

Tinnitus questions	Interpretation/s and discussion
What side is affected?	Right indicates more Yin involvement Left indicates more Yang involvement
Is the sound soft or louder?	Loud is generally an excess Soft/dim is generally a deficiency
Is the sound high pitched or low pitched?	High tones are an excess Lower tones are a deficiency

Questions 8, 9, and 10

Question 8 is about thirst, which we covered in eating and drinking. The Chinese practitioners I've worked with say this is newer thinking.

Question 9 is about previous illnesses, which you covered in the patient history.

Question 10 is about the causes of disease – what started it. But you covered that along the way too.

This page intentionally left blank.

CHAPTER 10
The Sixteen Modern Questions

The Sixteen Questions are an expansion of the Ten Traditional Questions. They cover taste, energy, sleep, menstrual issues, and emotional symptoms. I'll cover them by category rather than by the number, which combines a couple of them. Not to fear, you are generally only tested on the Ten Traditional Questions anyway.

This chapter starts at question 11, basically. No need to repeat the first ten, as they are the same in this list.

TASTE

This is about problems of being able to taste and also about predominant tastes a patient might have in their mouth either intermittently or constantly.

Taste	Interpretation/s and discussion
Bland	Nothing seems to have flavor or everything tastes the same. Sp/St Qi deficiency can cause this manifestation.
Sweet taste in the mouth	Sp/St damp heat
Acid regurgitation taste in the mouth	Heat in Lv and/or St.
Sour taste in the mouth	Food retention Smell the patient's breath. Often smells like sour milk, similar to what you sometimes smell on babies.

Bitter taste in the mouth	• St heat Look for red tongue with yellow coat, large fast pulse, voracious appetite. • Gb excess Irritable, distended feeling in hypochondria, pain in Gb channel
Salty taste in the mouth	• Ki deficiency • Cold
Metallic taste in the mouth	Think Lung dysfunction of some kind first, but can also signal an endocrine disorder.

ENERGY LEVEL

This one is kind of a duh. Low energy is Qi deficiency. To get more specific, ask if energy is low all the time or often seems that energy flags at certain times of the day.

If energy is low all the time, you might find that this patient has a Qi and/or Blood deficiency. If energy is low at certain times of the day, look at when then compare that to the bioclock below.

For example, I've had a lot of patients who reported flagging energy around 2-3 in the afternoon, in the middle of what would be the Small Intestine time period on the bioclock. When I ask, most of them say it's after they have had either a raw salad or something with bread in it (sandwich, burger, pasta, etc).

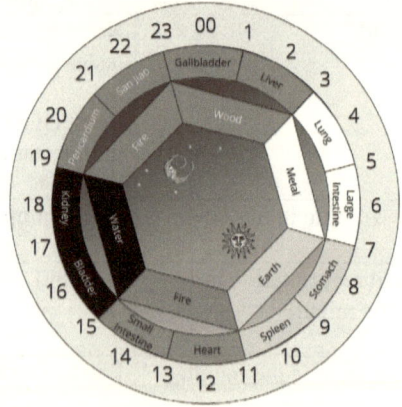

This often indicates a Spleen deficiency. The Small Intestine is the food processor and interacts with the Spleen to separate the turbid from the pure. When the Spleen is already weak, this puts further strain on that system, which causes the overall energy of the body to tank.

I live in Mexico. The way our building was wired would send an electrical inspector screaming down the block. Everything magically works somehow, but it's marginal on occasion. If my refrigerator is running and I plug in my electric teakettle, for instance, I can hear the refrigerator's electrical noise fall and the lights dim.

This is kind of like the Spleen when it's already deficient. Things are humming along functionally-ish then the Small Intestine starts knocking on its' door with a further work load and that causes the power drop. . . and the desire for an afternoon nap or an afternoon dose of caffeine.

And a note on caffeine. This will "fix" the problem temporarily, but can also cause sleep problems later in the evening. If your patient is band aid fixing their Spleen Qi deficiency and bad diet choices with caffeine, this is not a sustainable solution. This will backfire eventually. That's where you come in, Acupuncturist and Lifestyle Coach. Help them fix that noise!

Sleep

Sleep is another very important topic. This is what normal would look like.

Yang Qi is the component that is responsible for sleeping and waking. When all is well and in harmony, Yang Qi emerges around the eyes in the morning when you wake then circulates primarily in the superficial areas of the body so you can move around and get stuff done during your day. In the evening around bedtime the Yang Qi moves into the interior into the

Blood level and you fall asleep. This is why you get a little colder at night and often want to cover up – the Yang Qi isn't so active and doesn't warm your skin as much. This also means that at night you don't have a lot of defensive Qi on the surface, so it's easier to get sick at night.

But a lot of people have difficulty sleeping because the Yang Qi pattern gets "broken" for some reason. Why? There are about a billion reasons, so I'm not covering this in detail here. That will come later on in your educational process.

In the meantime, know that insomnia (sleep difficulties) come in several fun flavors.

Insomnia	Interpretation/s and discussion
Trouble falling asleep	Can't stop the monkey mind from chattering away, which keeps the patient awake. Often come along with a lot of vivid dreams, palpitations, night sweats, and low back soreness. Can be a Heart Kidney disharmony.
Sleeps very lightly	Wakes easily. Can be a sign of PTSD, as this comes along with hypervigilence, but can also signal a Heart/Spleen deficiency (sleeps lightly, palpitations, poor appetite, pale tongue).
Trouble staying asleep	Go to sleep easily, but wake in the middle of the night and have a hard time getting back to sleep. Pay attention to when the patient wakes and compare it to the ever so handy bioclock on page 94. Waking between 2 and 3 is really common and often comes with Lv disharmony. I'm an asthmatic and often wake between 3 and 5 – the Lung hours. Kidney Yang xu patients will often have diarrhea during the Large Intestine hours.

Restless sleep	Can be a Ht disharmony of some kind, heat (excess or deficient) in the interior, exterior heat, and more. Restless sleep with tossing, turning, belching, abdominal distention, and a tongue with a bean curd coating is food retention. St meridian has a branch going to the Ht, so dysfunction in the St will impact the Ht.
Sleeping too much	10+ hours of sleep desired per day. Can be a sign of depression. Too much sleep will actually make a body tired. It scatters the Qi when it is excessive, causes Qi deficiency and lethargy. Dampness, which blocks the dispersal of Qi and keeps Sp Qi from controlling the extremeties, can also cause sleepiness and heavy sensations. Blocked Sp Yang or deficient Sp Qi can be the cause.

Ask how long patients sleep. This can be affected strongly by PTSD (post traumatic stress disorder) of all kinds. Sleep circuits seem to get disturbed.

Asking if patients feel rested upon waking is a good indicator of the quality of sleep.

Vivid dreaming can also have a range of implications.

And of course, poor sleep can cause all kinds of health problems that need to be addressed as well.

DISEASES SPECIFIC TO WOMEN

By now you're probably picking up the general pattern of questions: how long have you had this, did it start after some event or other health condition, is there pain and where, what makes this better or worse, etc.

In addition to the usuals, you want to know some specific stuff about gynecological issues.
- Is there pain with your period?
    - Is the pain better with cold or heat?
- What is your period like?
    - What is the color of your bloods?
    - How much bleeding during your period is there?
    - Is the smell strong?
    - Do you have clots in the bloods?

Here is the short list of things you could see in clinic.

Menstrual problems	Interpretation/s and discussion
Early menstrual disorder	Period comes more often than every 28 days – usually 8-9 days ahead of time. Patients will often have heavy bleeding with lots of blood. Possible causes: • Blood heat • Sp Qi xu and unable to hold blood • Other Qi xu
Late menstrual disorder	Very long cycle – 8-9 days past the usual 28 days. Often has abdominal pain related to periods. Possible causes: • Blood deficiency • Cold contraction in the uterus
Irregular menstrual disorder	Possible causes: • Liver Qi stagnation

Short period	Shortened cycle, just a couple of days instead of the usual 5. • Blood heat (excess): short cycle, profuse bleeding, thick blood, fresh red in color. • Qi xu (deficiency): Lighter color, not as thick.
Amenorrhea	This is no period for 3 months or longer. Look for pale symptoms and other Blood xu signs. Possible causes: • Qi and/or Blood deficiency
Uterine bleeding	This means bleeding when there shouldn't be any. There are a myriad of reasons for this. You'll get more later.
Lower abdominal pain (usually dull) either before, during or after period	• Pain *after* the period is often a deficiency of Qi, Kidney, or Blood. • If pain *before* period, probably Lv Qi stagnation with Blood stasis. Pain is usually fixed at night. • Pain *during* the period is usually Qi and Blood stagnations combined. • If *after trauma* (i.e., car wreck where the seatbelt connects with the lower ab), or after surgery, could be Blood stasis. Generally a fixed pain.
Scanty, pale menses	Very low amount, color is like water color – very pale and watery. • Blood deficiency

Not to worry. You'll get way more gynecology during your education, probably in acupuncture, herbal, and western medicine studies and most likely several times over. This is an important topic, but it's not your only chance to get the information.

EMOTIONAL SYMPTOMS

Review the information about the seven emotions and the pathologies therein. Ask questions accordingly.

For whatever reason, different practitioners seem to draw different populations. Some practitioners do this on purpose. A friend of mine stood up at a business networking meeting one afternoon and announced she was looking for patients who had been diagnosed with cancer and were in the middle of chemotherapy. Suddenly she was swamped with this patient population.

Almost all of us get pain patients like crazy (so you should definitely get good at treating that), but some of us just seem to collect a certain patient population without even advertising for it. Another acupuncture colleague seems to attract autoimmune patients. One more gets geriatric patients. I seem to attract psycho emotional patients. I get a lot of stressed out patients, people with anxiety and/or depression, insomniacs (often the chief complaint, but usually fueled by anxiety and Heart/Liver issues), and bipolar folks.

This isn't on your boards, and you aren't likely to be tested on it unless you are taking specific classes about treating emotions later on, but I thought I'd share my "starter pack" questions to get people talking about their emotional stuff.

Cat's questions	Why I ask this
What's your predominant emotion when nothing special is going on?	To get a sense of how the patient *feels* most of the time.
Are you irritable or angry a lot?	Indicates possible internal heat and/or Lv issues.
Do you feel sad or hopeless frequently?	Indicates possible Qi or Blood stagnation/stasis, depression.

So you have mood swings?	Can indicate Qi stagnation, *might* hint at bipolar disorder
Would your partner, significant other, spouse agree with your answers?	OK, I feel pretty chill most of the time... I think... but I'm a long term Liver Qi stagnation poster child, so my spouse would disagree with my perception of my chillness. People often aren't able to see objectively, so can have a skewed view of their own emotional landscape. But they can almost always tell you exactly how their family sees them.
What is your go-to emotion when things get stressful in your life?	Some people get angry (that's me) and frustrated. Some people shut down and disconnect. That tells you what the underlying emotion is just below the surface.
Do you self-medicate with alcohol or other substances?	See what I did there? That opens the door for conversations about addictive behavior, regardless of the substance.*

*Fun thing to know: self-soothing with food, drugs (illicit or prescribed), alcohol, cigarettes, caffeine, etc. points to addictive behavior patterns. That's about our own chemical production of dopamine and we are all addicted to that! But some people can't feel the happy enough on their own, so they add artificial dopamine sources to feel better. This doesn't mean the patient is an addict, but does point to an emotional imbalance. *Way* more about this later on.

This is by no means an exhaustive discussion on emotions. Maciocia wrote a whole book on it, for Pete's sake! As a very general rule of thumb, you'll discover that depression is often fueled by deficiency of Qi and Qi stagnation and is frequently Liver related. If the Qi isn't flowing smoothly, the Shen isn't able to flow smoothly either. Anxiousness is often Heart and

Liver related with Liver Qi stagnation, Liver fire, and a "floating" Shen that can't rest. Irritation is generally heat-related in some way. People with a bipolar diagnosis often have combinations of stagnation and heat. ADD/ADHD folks often have Liver wind and Liver Yang rising.

Section 4:
Pulse Diagnosis

You'll learn *about* pulse diagnosis here, but you aren't going to actually *learn* it without putting your fingers on an awful lot of wrists. Pulse diagnosis is like muscle memory. You do it enough and your fingers, your brain, and your intuition start communicating to give you truly valuable information about your patient.

What you *will* learn here are the names and characteristics of each pulse, which you will need to know for many, many tests and for clinical experience approximately forever.

Left it blank on purpose. Don't freak out.

Chapter 11
Pulse Diagnosis Basics

Pulse Diagnosis Introduction

Almost every student I've ever taught or known (myself included) was intimidated by pulse diagnosis. Why? Because it's a hard skill to learn! Using the pulse to interpret the health of a client is a very old art form and takes years to master.

Lemme tell you. When I was in the beginning of my 2nd year in school, I took an advanced pulse seminar. I didn't really think I was ready for it at the time, but needed the extra hour on my schedule. I found myself in the seminar with people two and three years ahead of me in school. To my surprise, they had the same feelings of intimidation and sense of confusion that I had about pulses even after spending more years in student clinic than I had.

The seminar turned out to be one of the best things I did in school. It took a lot of the confusion and intimidation out of the mix and helped me relax about it. After that I found my pulse taking was easier and I wasn't so hard on myself about getting it wrong.

This section on pulses will give you the basics foundation to work with, starting you on the path to becoming conversant in pulses. To really get great you have to work at it, take a lot of pulses, and most importantly of all, learn to trust your own instincts about what you feel.

Remember that two people feeling the same pulse may have different descriptions of that pulse. One person may say it's wiry and the next says it's slippery. Can they both be right?

Quite possibly so. This is a very subjective experience! As you're learning to take pulses you'll make your life a lot simpler and will feel less insecure about what you feel if you just accept this as a fact:

Different people will get different findings from the same pulse.

Remember too that the pulse is an excellent way to find out what's happening in the body. You can use what you feel and your analysis of that to drive your inquiry (the questions you ask your patient) and may very well get much more information than you would just by sitting and asking the diagnostic questions we covered in the previous chapters.

But the pulse isn't the *only* way to get information, nor is it your only diagnostic tool. Combine the pulse findings with questions/answers from the patient interview, tongue diagnosis, points that are tender on the body, etc. in order to form your pattern differentiations and treatment plans.

The uber-basics

When you get what a pulse is down to the very basic components, you find that it's not dissimilar from any other kind of fluid pumping system. If you've ever had a fish tank, worked on the water pump in your car, or had a backyard pond with a pump, this will sound very familiar.

The whole heart system is basically three mechanical parts:
- Pump – the heart itself
- Fluid – the blood
- Tubes – the blood vessels

That's a really simplified version of the whole circulatory system! When you are feeling the pulse you are feeling how the fluid that is pumping through the tubes is interacting with the interior conditions – the emotions, the internal organs, sensations of pain, etc.

The takeaway here is:
1) It's very subjective
2) Everyone struggles with it – don't be unnecessarily hard on yourself!
3) It takes a long time to learn it well
4) Feel an awful lot of pulses. Make notes about what you feel, even if you don't remember all of the "correct" pulse terms when you're doing it.

If you can pick up three qualities of the pulse, celebrate! That's more information about your patient than you had a second ago.

Ok, that said, let's jump into this.

Pulse Basics – Beyond Uber-basics

Did you know that the classic method of taking the pulse at the wrist was not always the norm? True story. There used to be eight common pulse points around the body – at the temples, carotid pulse, abdominal pulse, pulse on the top of the foot, at the groin, and a few more that have largely been lost in time for most of us. Why did it change? Blame Confucius. His philosophies emphasized personal and social morality, justice, sincerity and a lot of very good things. . . but his prudishness is the reason why it became socially *un*acceptable to take pulses around the body. Chinese docs suddenly had to use nothing more than wrist points to figure out the pump and fluid's interaction with the interior of the body.

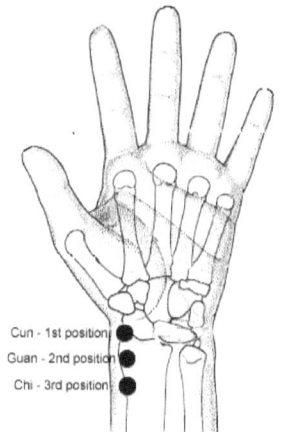
Cun - 1st position
Guan - 2nd position
Chi - 3rd position

So now, here we are limited to three tiny points on each wrist. Thanks a lot, Confucius.

The pulse points
Obviously, you need to know what those points are.

Pulse points	Brief discussion
Cun	This is the 1st position and it is the closest to the wrist crease.

"Cun" refers to a small unit of measure and is sometimes translated as inch. |
| Guan | This is the 2nd position of the three, lying in between the 1st and 3rd positions.

"Guan" means gate or barr. This refers to its' position in relation to the other two. |
| Chi | This is the 3rd position, the most distal from the wrist crease.

Chi means a larger unit of measure and is sometimes translated as "foot" or "cubit" if you want to get really old school about it. |

What the positions represent on either side
I'm giving you the most common TCM interpretations of the positions. There are many others and there is no right and no wrong. Old school texts will tell you to pick a method that works and go with it.

BUT, since you are just learning and since this is tested on most national boards, learn these for now. You can branch out later.

Left wrist	Position	Right wrist
Heart	Cun – 1st position	Lung
Liver/Gallbladder	Guan – 2nd position	Spleen/Stomach
Kidney Yang, lower abdomen, Mingmen	Chi – 3rd position	Kidney Yin, lower abdomen, Shen

Finding the pulse points

To accurately read the pulse you need to put your fingers in the right spot. A lot of texts will start by saying something like "place your *middle finger (Guan, 2nd position) beside and proximal to the styloid process of the radius on the radial artery*…"

You should probably memorize that language. I've seen it on a lot of tests. But I don't find it to be a very reliable method of placing your fingers down in the right spot on the radial arteries on the wrists. Here's what I learned from one of my professors:

1. Have the patient's lay both hands and lower arms on the table across from you with the lateral edge of the arm on the table and the medial edge of the arm facing up toward the ceiling like this → and with both palms facing their chest.

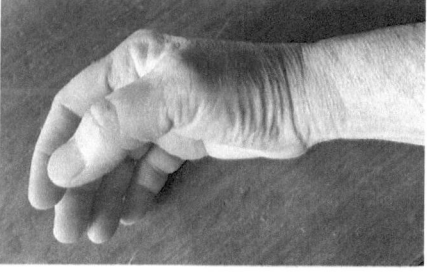

This allows you to reach comfortably without crimping your own wrists, which will mess with your ability to feel the pulse fully. This also keeps the patient's wrists at about the level of the heart, which is ideal for pulse taking.

2. Where exactly do you put your fingers?
    a. Rest *the tip* of your index finger just proximal to the crease of the wrist on the radial artery. There is a little depression right there. You might have the patient curl their wrist inward toward the inside of the forearm (palm-ward) if you want to feel this depression a little easier. This little divot is right around the LU 9 acupuncture point on the radial side of the wrist.

    b. Drop *the tip* of your middle finger down right next to that and you should find that this fingertip falls just on the proximal side of the styloid process of the wrist.

    c. Drop *the tip* of your ringer finger down right next to the middle finger. If you slide your ring finger proximally a little big you should feel the edge of the large brachioradialis muscle. You should be just distal to the edge of that muscle.

This is true for just about everyone, but we all have different body sizes. You might have to wiggle your 2nd and 3rd finger around a bit to find the ideal spot on a bigger or smaller person.

Notice I said you feel the pulse with the *tip* of your fingers. This is generally the most sensitive part of the fingers, so that's what you want to use. When you are asked about this on a test, this is the right answer.

But if you are a guitar player or if you have had carpal tunnel or anything else that might truncate sensation in the fingertips, you might have to use the finger pads. I was told that I had to give up playing guitar if I ever wanted to be really good at pulses. So I quit playing and I've regretted it since. Don't do it. Compensate in other ways.

Funky Pulse Positions

About 30% of the population has some non-normal anatomical characteristics. Some of these affect the pulse positions. These are congenital and are considered normal, *but* if you discover you cannot find the pulse where you expect it to be on the wrist and your patient is obviously alive and animate, look in these places.(Or wear garlic – vampires, you know.)

- Opposite Gate Pulse (fan guan mai in Chinese/Pinyin) – patient's radial artery runs on the dorsal side of the arm. Rare, but it happens.

- Oblique Flying Pulse (xie fei mai) – patient's radial artery goes at an oblique angle from 3rd position to 1st position, going diagonally towards the dorsal side. You might find the 1st position, but 2nd and 3rd will be toward the dorsal side of the wrist in a diagonal line.

(Maciocia says when you encounter these you should really take pulses at alternate points on the body to get the reading these positions would normally indicate. Unfortunately, he failed to elaborate and tell us where these were!)

How long to take the pulse

For a minute or two. This gives you the opportunity to feel for repetitive patterns, irregularities, and to do a pulse count also (for the biomed portion of your charting).

How deep to press
There are three depths to feel for.

Depth	Brief discussion
Superficial	This is also called "lifting." You are just resting your fingers on the pulse points and not pressing deeply at all. This allows you to feel for the superficial pulses that indicate that a disease is in the exterior region of the body.
Medium	Also called "searching." You are pressing with medium pressure on the pulse points so you can feel the quality of the blood going through the vessels.
Deep	Also called "pressing." This is the deepest pressure. You are almost squishing the vessel pretty firmly to see if there is any pushback in the pulse, which indicates good root or good basic Qi.

Best time to take the pulse
This is an academic discussion because chances are good you aren't going to have the opportunity to do this, but the best time to take the pulse is technically early in the morning before the patient gets out of bed.

Since changes are good you can't do that, let the patient sit and rest for a while before taking the pulse.

Ideal posture
This is also academic, but you could have test questions on this. My favorite posture is sitting across a desk or table from the client and having them put their wrists in the position as described above. It's comfortable, doesn't stress the patient's arms or yours, and you can feel both wrists at the same time this way.

- Wrist should be on about the same level as the heart.
- Sitting or lying down is fine. Not standing up.

Method for pulse taking

1. Feel with all 3 fingers on both sides simultaneously. This allows you to feel the overall pulse quality and character before moving on to the character/quality of the individual positions.

    a. Feel all 3 depths – superficial, medium, and deep.
    b. Push – move fingers laterally side to side in each position to feel around the pulse and determine its shape and qualities.
    c. Roll – move fingers proximal to distal in each position to determine short, long, moving (and to read pulse in child aged 1 year of less).
    d. Feel for speed of the pulse.
    e. Feel for rhythm. Feel for 50 beats in order to determine rhythm or arrhythmia.

2. Feel the individual positions on each side of the body. Be sure to feel at all 3 depths for each individual position also, repeating the stuff above .

An Ideal Pulse

Now that you have your patient positioned and you're ready to take the pulses. . . what exactly are you feeling for? Let's explore the ideal pulse in a healthy patient first so you can compare that to the pathological pulses.

Ideal pulse characteristics	Brief discussion
Has root	Root can mean two things. You're feeling for both of them. • Can refer to the chi or 3rd pulse position Pulse here should be strong, as this is the Kidney position and the root of our whole constitution. • Can refer to the deepest level of the pulse as you press from the surface of the skin downward in a vertical motion. You are pressing deeply so that the vessel is pretty squished but not quite flat. If you press down deeply and the pulse still pushes back so that you can feel the pulse, this is good root.
Has good Stomach Qi	This is about as subjective as it gets! This is the Goldilocks of pulses – not too fast, not too slow, not to weak, not too strong, but *just* right. This shows that the constitution is moderate and working well. The center of everything, the Earth, the Spleen and Stomach, are in harmony.
Has good Shen	Good stability, good rate of speed, good volume of blood in the vessels.
Matches the season of the year	• Spring: Pulse is wirier, but still moderate with moderate tension in the vascular system. Like in the environment when Spring is the time where things expand, so does the body. There is more warmth and movement in the blood compared to the contraction of winter.

	• Summer: Pulse surges a little, but isn't hurried. A bit more superficial than other seasons. The heat of the season is being reflected inside and the heat comes to the surface a little. A surging pulse is also called a 'hooked' pulse. Think of the shape of an ocean wave as it comes onto the shore. There's a surge of energy pushing it into a wave shape, but not enough to sustain it to the end, so you get the curl of the wave and then the quick collapse of the energy. • Autumn: Pulse feels moderate again, perhaps slightly choppy. • Winter: Pulses, like the energy of the environment, goes inward slightly and will be a little deeper.
Matches in position	Evenly distributed throughout the positions.

How fast should the pulse be?

If you've had biomedical training, you will remember that a 'normal' pulse speed is **between 60 and 90bpm**. Since clocks and watches with sweeping second hands are a fairly recent invention, traditional docs in China had to do things differently.

Chinese medicine docs would match their breath to the patient's breath speed and depth, then feel the number of beats. Normal is considered to be **4 heart beats to 1 inhale/exhale cycle**.

This page intentionally left blank.

Chapter 12:
Pathological Pulses

Now that you have a familiarity with positioning, what the positions mean, and have a working description of ideal pulses, it's time to talk pathologies.

There are several categories of pathological pulses with a number of individual pulses in each category for a grand total of about 28 different pulses. Some books have a few more, like the "Strange Pulses," but they are rare to encounter. That's a lot of pulses. I'll lay each category of pulses out in a chart and will mark the ones you need to know for testing purposes.

The categories are: superficial, rapid, deficient, excess, some combinations of these, and the strange pulses.

Superficial Pulses

Superficial or floating pulses usually indicate an *exterior* problem. In special cases it may indicate the yang floating up – and creating a false shen, but by and large, it's an exterior condition.

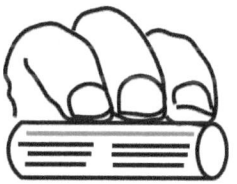

See the bad, out of proportion diagram to the right? This red line is where you will find this pulse. *Touch very lightly* (also called "lifting technique" in order to feel this pulse or you will squish it and miss is.

Remember, as a general rule, cold conditions are indicated by slow pulses while heat conditions will have a fast pulse. Also, if it's **bold** below make a special note of that. Likely to be quizzed on that.

Name	Description	Indications
Superficial Floating *Chinese:* *Fu*	Pulse has most strength at uppermost level and can be felt with only slight touch. Can feel w/light touch Grows faint on hard pressure.	• External Pathogen Circulation of qi and blood is focused in the body's surface to deal with external agent. Internal circulation temperature is sacrificed to focus on elimination of the pathogen, in an attempt to keep it from moving deeper. • Deficiency Debilitated pts may have feeble, floating pulse: inability to retain Qi and Yang in interior due to deficiency of vital organs.
Surging Overflowing Flooding *Chinese:* *Hong*	Broad, large, forceful Like a wave with a forceful rise, but a gradual decline See the bad drawing? You are catching the top of the wave as it begins to dissipate.	• Excess heat Force of pulse is pathological. Gradual decline at the end indicates the heat syndrome. This is due to Qi excess not a fluid excess, despite the name.
Soft Soggy *Chinese:* *Ru*	Superficial, thready, w/o strength. Thin, soft. With a light touch, feels like a thread floating on water. When you press more deeply, feels faint.	• Deficiency Progressed states of disease with Xu of Qi, Yin and Blood, all of which allow the Yang to float. If the pulse disappears when you press, the

		yang is expiring.
		• Dampness
		Note: because it feels easily movable (like thread floating), tends to indicate SP Qi xu w/accumulation of dampness.
Scattered *Chinese:* *San* **Crisis pulse!**	Superficial, scattered, indistinct irregular without root. Hardly perceptible. Diffuses on a light touch, feels faint when you press heavily. This is a large, floating, weak pulse. Vessel wall is very thin, seems to scatter like powder when you touch it. It's even hard to count the beats.	• Depletion of Yuan Qi! Hence the crisis. Note: These are cases where patients are critically ill, are hospitalized or sent home to die; diagnosis is usually well-established. Pulse says only that patient is severely ill.
Hollow *Chinese:* *Kou*	Superficial, large, empty (like stalk of green onion). Feels floating, large, soft, hollow (like a drinking straw or green onion) Feels wide and distinct when you feel from one side of the vessel to the other. Superficial: can feel it lightly Mid level: *barely* there Deep level: can feel it lightly	• Blood loss, Blood xu • Yin xu "Green onion" feel means there is some Qi flow at the surface of the vessel, but not so much in the blood level. Researchers at Beijing University say this is due to hemorrhagic conditions like severe blood loss or internal bleeding. Can also indicate a loss of essence.

Leather Tympanic *Chinese:* Ge	Wiry, fast, superficial, without root, feels empty inside, like the head of a drum. Thin wall Normal wall Thick wall Wide from one side of the vessel to the other, vessel wall will feel thick.	• Essence xu • Blood xu You find this in older men a lot. If you see it in another age bracket can indicate cocaine use, multiple personality disorders, ritual abuse and more.
Superficial Pulse combinations to know		
Floating + Tight	External cold. You might also see chills and fever, aversion to cold, tongue pale with thin white coat, no sweating, and/or clear watery nasal discharge.	
Floating + fast	External heat. You might also see headache, nasal discharge yellow/sticky, sweating, chills and fever (but more fever than chills).	
Superficial + slowed down	External deficiency. An external invasion of some kind + a deficiency in the constitution. With an exterior + deficiency you will see sweating of a wimpy nature that doesn't help expel the pathogen. Might also have chills and a fever.	
Superficial + slippery	**Exterior syndrome with phlegm/damp retention.** Superficial = exterior, slippery = phlegm/damp	

Deep Pulses

Deep pulses are felt by pressing heavily all the way to the organ depth, or at least half way down. Deep and sinking pulses indicate an *interior or chronic* (prolonged) problem. If the pulse is strong and deep this indicates an internal excess. If the pulse is weak and deep, it signals an internal deficiency.

And of course, remember that slow indicates cold while fast indicates heat. Pay special attention to anything **bolded**!

Name	Description	Indications
Deep Sinking Chinese: Chen	Strongest at the lowest level. Requires deep pressure to feel well. Can only be felt by pressing hard.	• Internal syndrome • Circulation of Qi and Blood from internal viscera to the surface is weak Note: Circulation in this case is confined to the interior as the body attempts to deal with a serious disorder threatening the internal organs.
Hidden Chinese: Fu	Can only be felt by pressing to the bone. Located even deeper than the sinking pulse. Note: Extreme pulse. Can barely detect the pulse except with deep pressure to or near the level of the bone. You might get a sense that the pulse is hidden in the muscles or perhaps	• Closing syndrome (in this case, pulse closes too) • Syncope (loss of consciousness) • Extreme pain Note 1: Conditions such as LOC (loss of consciousness) and severe pain can be

	resting on the surface of the bone	easily determined w/o taking pulse. Note 2: There are two kinds of loss consciousness—closing and opening syndromes. Note 3: This is a form of protection to keep the Shen inside.
Firm Confined *Chinese:* *Lao*	Full, large, wiry and long Is a form of hidden pulse. Opposite of leathery. Can also be very deep, wiry, usually long and strong. One final description: Deep, taut, wiry, long, large, forceful. Combined together. Wiry refers to the feel of a guitar string – tight and hard and resistant to pressure.	• Cold • Internal excess • Shan disorder (hernia) • Mass of some kind It's unusual to find this pulse.
Weak Frail *Chinese:* *Ruo*	Feels Deep, thready, w/o strength (soft) Cannot feel this pulse superficially!	• Qi deficiency and Blood deficiency Usually from a long term condition. Occurs when the Qi cannot support the pulse and there isn't enough blood to make the pulse strong. Note 1: Usually indicates weakness of SP Qi leading to deficiency of both qi and blood.

		Note 2: Similar to fine pulse, but softer in quality
		Note 3: Is basically the opposite of the replete (shi) pulse.

Deep Pulse combinations to know	
Deep + slow	**Internal cold.** Can be excess or xu, depending on how strongly it hits your fingertip, on how long its' been going on. Could have also just ingested something cold. Look at the tongue – swollen w/teeth marks, and look for other cold confirming signs.
Deep + thin	**Internal condition and deficiency, usually of Yin or Blood.** Thin is distinct, no matter where located. Shape should be very clear. Thin is under the finger like a thread. This pulse would probably be fast— generally a yin deficiency or blood deficiency.
Deep + slowed down	**Internal condition + damp/deficiency** Spleen Qi xu will have this type of pulse. Damp is sticky and slows everything down.
Deep + slippery	**Interior condition + dampness.**

SLOW PULSES

A slow pulse is usually less than 60bpm – or less than one breath for every 4 pulse beats. Exceptions include athletes in great shape who may have much lower pulse than non-athletes.

Slow pulses *usually* indicate cold conditions…*however*, **choppy does *not* indicate cold.** Pay special attention to anything **bolded**!

Name	Description	Indications

Slow
 	
Chinese: Chi
	Pulse is less than 60 bpm (usually 40-60 bpm), or less than 4 pulse beats per breath.	• Cold syndrome
		  o Yang xu = empty cold - slow, weak and deep.
		  o Yin excess = full cold – slow and strong
		
		Must be interpreted in light of other diagnostic info since slow pulse could be due to other reasons (like very fit athletes).

Slowed – down Relaxed Loose Moderate *Chinese:* Huan	When you measure with a clock or by beats/breath, it doesn't fall into the *slow* category, but the pulse *feels* sluggish to you. There is diminished tension in pulse. Normal in depth, speed, strength, width.	• Dampness • Phlegm • Spleen Qi xu. Look for greasy tongue coating, perhaps MJ discomfort to support your suspicion. Note: Pulse has a softness/looseness due to weakness of Qi + obstructing effect of damp. Differs from phlegm-damp in that it has no solidity.
Choppy Uneven	Pulse is uneven and *rough* (like scraping down bamboo	• Qi stagnation • Blood deficiency

Hesitant *Chinese:* *Se*	or a branch with a lot of knots with a knife). Also described in texts as "coming and going choppily w/small, fine, slow, joggling tempo." Usually found in the deep areas, but might be in middle/searching area. Feel for brief hesitations or interruptions in movement. Takeaway: this is not a smooth pulse in any way.	You'll see this when the severity of blood disorder is great – will be quite forceless. • Blood stasis/stagnation You could see this in patients with arterio-sclerosis and in severe blood deficiency, but also in trauma victims who also have qi/blood stagnation • Essence deficiency • Phlegm retention • Food retention **NEVER indicates Cold!!** Know this!
Knotted *Chinese:* *Jie*	***Slow* pulse with irregular missed beats.** This is a key point to know for the test! Pulse seems to miss a beat w/o an apparent pattern	• Yin excess • Cold phlegm • Blood stasis • Qi stagnation • Blockage • Obstruction Note: Can indicate coronary artery disease when accompanied by chest pain. Note 2: Circulation could be blocked by phlegm, cold, tumors or any number of pathogens. It can occur in deficiencies when Qi and Blood are insufficient to fill the channels so that pathogens fill in the gap and cause the arrhythmia

RAPID PULSES

Rapid pulses are 5 beats per breath or more. From a biomedical perspective, a pulse that is too fast is 90-140 bpm. Anything higher than that means the heart could slide into tachycardia and arrest. Call 911!

Rapid pulses indicate heat conditions! If it's in **bold**, know it.

Name	Description	Indications
Rapid **Fast** *Chinese:* *Shuo*	90+ bpm or 5+ beats per respiratory	• Heat Syndrome Bit more rapid than normal, usually occurs only when serious illness, when there is fever. • Yang Excess: Pulse is strong and rapid • Yin Deficiency: Thin, fast, weak NOTE: Pulse can become rapid from activity prior to pulse taking. Don't jump to the conclusion of heat without other supporting evidence!
Abrupt Hasty Running Hurried *Chinese:* *Cu*	Hurried, rapid, with irregular/irregular* missed beats (jie mai pulse). Also described in some texts as hasty and rapid with irregular intermittence. Irregular, missed, fast. Similar to knotted. Sometimes described as a man running and stumbling in old texts.	• Excessive Yang heat • Qi and blood stagnation • Phlegm retention • Food retention Note: this is like an excess version of knotted pulse. Rapidity indicates heat and irregular indicates blockage

	*Irregular/irregular means that there are missed/skipped heart beats, but there is no pattern to it. Better prognosis when the irregularity occurs at regular intervals.	caused by stagnation and/or accumulation.
NOTE about Hasty pulse: Can signal a misfire of the heart's AV node. The more frequent the miss, the more likely there is a biomedical cardiopathology. I suggest you use biomedical terminology in your charts for this one. You are likely to need to refer the patient out to a cardiologist. Use med-speak when you communicate around these issues and with these folks so you are taken seriously. Your patient's life might be on the line here.		
Swift *Chinese:* *Ji* **Crisis pulse!**	Somewhere around 120 – 140 bpm or 7 beats per breath cycle. Feels hasty and swift. Palpitations	• Depletion of Yuan Qi Pulse is so rapid (twice as fast as normal) that it is easily detected. The acute febrile disease involves an easily measured high temperature, usually pathology can be found in testing. Consumptive conditions w/such high pulse are generally under emergency medical care.
Moving Spinning bean *Chinese:* *Dong*	Short, slippery, fast, forceful. Combination of short, tight, slippery, rapid pulses. Felt in only *one* position, not all. Also described as "incomplete, without a head or tail, like a bean." You cannot feel this easily, I was told…and yet I have. Twice.	• Pain • Fright

DEFICIENT PULSES

Deficient pulses are also called "empty" or "vacuous" pulses. They can feel large, but they yield under pressure easily and you will find no force in these pulses. Lack of force is the primary distinction here. No big surprise, but these indicate deficient conditions. Pay special attention to anything in **bold** below.

Name	Description	Indications
Empty Deficiency *Chinese:* Xu	**Forceless on the three regions at all 3 levels of pressure** (key point for this pulse). Feels feeble and void. Easy pulse to mistake. Pay attention to the key point bolded above.	• Deficiency syndrome Similar to weak, fine, faint pulses. Occurs when deficiency of blood is more severe than in weak/fine pulses, but not so deficient as the faint pulse. So on a scale of severity, least to most severe: 1) weak, 2) fine, 3) empty/deficient, 4) faint.
Minute Feeble Faint *Chinese:* Wei **Crisis pulse!**	Extremely thin/thready and soft; scarcely perceptible. Weaker than the thready pulse. Feels this way on all levels, all pressures.	• Yin deficiency • Yang deficiency • Qi deficiency • Xue deficiency Extreme exhaustion is obvious to both patient and doc. Pulse lacks substance, volume, strength; exhaustion of body essences. Prognosis is very bad.
Thready Thin Fine *Chinese:* Xi	Fine thread. **Very distinct and clear.** Can be strong but slender. Can feel at all depths/levels No kidding: it feels like a literal thread from one side	• Deficiency due to overstrain and stress • Yin deficiency • Blood deficiency • Qi deficiency • Dampness

	of the vessel to the other. You can feel it at all 3 depths.	• Essence deficiency due to chronic illness
Intermittent Regularly intermittent Chinese: Dai	Regularly irregular – pulse seems to miss a beat or pause at predictable intervals and with definite pattern. A slow pulse. *This is the only regular irregular pulse!*	• Exhaustion of the organs • Trauma (accident) Usually only see in cases where patient is hospitalized or in advanced disease stage. Example: serious heart disease due to deficiency/ blockage, blood stasis/phlegm.

Note on Intermittent pulses
The more frequent the missed beat, the more serious the case – if the miss is every 4 beats, refer to a western doc!

Sometimes the beat isn't *missed*, but the intensity of the beats changes – press deeper to see if the beat is still missed.

If the amplitude comes and goes it means that the mitochondria aren't recovering quickly in the system and that the system is therefore somewhat fatigued. This is a heart Qi deficiency. Usually only see this in elderly folks. Can also be blood stasis anywhere in the body – this is the heart pumping against a stagnation (scar tissues, etc.) and fatiguing the heart.

Short* Chinese: Duan	Pulse with short extent. Short pulse seems to deteriorate from central pulse position towards the 2 adjacent pulse positions. Strikes the middle finger sharply, leaves quickly. *You can't feel a short pulse in all 3 positions. Despite what the text above says, you could also feel this in*	• Qi deficiency • Qi stagnation or blockage Contraction of Qi – usually Liver Qi stagnation

| | the 1st or 3rd positions, but if so you won't feel it in the others. | |

A note about short pulses:
Conditions within the body can affect the structure of the vessel itself (like in a short pulse the problem could be a ganglion cyst at the wrist affecting the shape of the vessel and thus the flow through it), or can affect how blood flows in the vessels. The latter might mean that Blood flow is impacted by stagnant Qi and that can mean that the qi is failing to move the blood so that the pulse positions are not filled. *Deficiency or stagnation are the primary reasons for a short pulse.*

EXCESS PULSES

Indicate excess conditions, obvs, and are also called full and replete pulses.

This is a forceful pulse felt in all three finger positions and at all three depths. The vessel itself feels full. It will give you the impression that it is long (you can move your 3rd finger proximally and you can still feel it in the artery), large (thick/wide from one side of the vessel to the other), and forceful. *Force is the primary distinction to an excessive pulse.*

If you think you are feeling this in an elderly person, press to the lowest depth and see if there's root. There probably won't be. This is likely to be a cardiac pathology.

As usual, if **it's bold** in the following table, pay particular attention to that.

Name	Description	Indications
Full Replete **Forceful** Excess *Chinese: Shi*	**Pulse can be felt strongly on all 3 levels.** Feels vigorous and forceful on both light and heavy pressure. Very strong.	• Excess heat Gives little info other than condition = excess. Use all other diagnostic skills to determine the nature of the excess. Generally, indicates you should not use tonification because this also indicates the body's resistance is undamaged.
Slippery Smooth Rolling *Chinese: Hua*	Described in classical texts as: *Smooth, like a row of pearls on a dish rolling past under your fingers or like beads rolling on a plate.* *Very regular and orderly, hitting the fingers one at a time.* Yeah, I don't roll like that. That makes no sense to me. Drum your fingers on the table like you are getting impatient. Feel how one hits at a time? The slippery pulse feels kind of like that, only you aren't moving your fingers.	• Dampness • Phlegm • Food retention • Pregnancy (often called "happy pulse" in China) While this pulse can be a normal condition it is often good confirmation of diagnosis of phlegm-damp accumulation. **Never indicates deficiency!**
Slippery Combination to know		
Slippery + fast	• **Damp heat** Damp is in the Middle Jiao, Sp can't metabolize water well, so generates damp which is sticky and leads to heat.	

	• **Phlegm heat/fire** Phlegm is primarily stored in the lungs but can also be present in the meridians. Phlegm is more condensed and sticky than just dampness. This is like dampness, but congealed by either heat cooking the excess liquid off or congealed by cold. Phlegm in the Lung is literal phlegm that can (eventually) be coughed out. Phlegm in the meridians is "invisible" phlegm. or it could be invisible phlegm. Invisible phlegm can cause Shen disturbance by blocking the easy flow of Qi and blood to and from the heart and brain and it can get blown around by an inner wind and cause a condition such as a stroke. Phlegm, literal or invisible can cause stagnation and blockage which can lead to an interior condition of fire. • **Food retention** Babies and kids get this a lot. Food retention means the food isn't moving in the digestive tract which generates internal heat and fevers.	
Tight Tense *Chinese:* *Jin*	Tight, forceful like a stretched rope or tightly stretched cord. Feels thicker than the Xian or Wiry pulse. Tight is the hardest – no flex Wiry – hard, but will still flex Slippery – soft and flexible	• Cold. Cold stretches and contracts, hence the tight tense pulse. Exterior cold will be more superficial, internal cold will be tight, slow. • Pain • Food retention Similar to wiry pulse, but not as long. While pain can easily be reported, cold is sometimes disguised by localized heat symptoms. This pulse can indicate either exterior or interior cold.

Long *Chinese:* *Chang*	Refers to the length of the pulse from one side of your fingertip to the other. Described in classics as: Straight/ beyond position Pulse w/long extent, prolonged stroke. *Can* show that the vessels are strong and flexible. In young people especially, can feel this pulse across all 3 finger positions at once. But can also reflect pathology →	• Excess Yang Qi • Heat Stringy quality indicates a level of tension, corresponds to a Lv syndrome. If patient has an acute disease, long pulse will occur when there is a strong confrontation between body resistance and pathogen.
Wiry Stringy Taut String taut Bowstring *Chinese:* *Xian*	Long, tense, stable and can be felt with different pressures. Taut, straight, long, **like violin string**. Feels straight and long, like musical string instrument. Hits all 3 fingers at the same time. Note: leathery pulse is superficial, feels similar, but wiry pulse is not a superficial pulse. *I think this feels like someone thwacking my fingertip hard and fast. Just sayin.'*	• Liver problem • Gallbladder problem (inflammation— alcohol and fried foods make it worse) • Pain • Phlegm • Malaria Similar to tense pulse, but longer, more tremulous. Severe pain can be easily reported, but wiry pulse confirms Lv and/or Gb as the point of disharmony.
Wiry Pulse combinations to know		
Wiry + Fast	Lv heat May have a bitter taste in the mouth and/or anger. Hepatitis patients have this pulse in the acute stage. Look	

	at the tongue: the sides will be red or you might see a red tongue, possibly with a yellow coat.
Wiry + Thin	Lv and Ki Yin deficiency Hypertension patients and arteriosclerosis patients can have this pulse. Hits the fingers hard and strong.

A quick chat about "Slippery"

What the heck makes the pulse "slippery?" What makes the feel of the drumming on the table or the pearls sliding across a plate or however you want to word that for yourself?

Basically: turbulence in the flow of blood caused by a partial obstruction of some kind. The obstruction could be cholesterol buildup (a form of phlegm, by the way), something anatomical that is pushing on the outside of the vessel wall (like a ganglion cyst at the wrist), or dampness making things sticky and impeding the smooth flow within the vessel.

In the illustration below you see the mirrored "hills" that represents a cholesterol buildup at the top and bottom of the vessel. See how the blood flow changes as a result of the partial blockage?

Something similar happens in flowing rivers. An unobstructed river flows smoothly. Put some big boulders in it and the flow is changed, causing swirls and eddies.

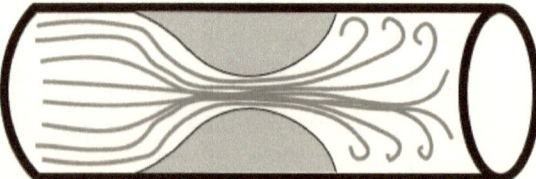

When you think of it like that, slippery takes on a whole new meaning. Slippery is often phlegm and/or damp resulting the impedances in the flow, but bear in mind that more than just damp or phlegm might cause this.

STRANGE AND DEATH PULSES

All you need to know for purposes of tests is that there are **10 strange pulses** indicating very severe conditions and **7 death pulses**. Both indicate dangerous conditions with poor prognosis—Yang is almost gone, Stomach qi almost gone. This dude is dead, man.

Fun side note
Some of the strange pulses have awesome names. Here are a few merely to entertain you:
- Circling Fish Pulse
- Leaking roof pulse
- Bird Pecking Pulse
- Swimming Shrimp Pulse
- Boiling Pot Pulse

This page intentionally left blank.

SECTION 4: PALPATION

OK, technically taking the pulse is a form of palpation, but this small section is about palpating the body and the channels. This is the super basic version of palpation. Learn the super basics now, but later in your education (may in school, maybe in CEUs you will need for your license later on) you will get more on palpating the body. Japanese acupuncture methods have a heavy focus on channel and point palpation. There is a whole school of thought about abdominal palpation. Wait on those for now.

This page intentionally left blank.

CHAPTER 13:
Palpation

Palpation is touching, pressing, and feeling the body in some way (and yes, that includes pulses). Make sure your hands are clean and as warm as you can make them before you palpate! Your patients will appreciate that.

PALPATING SKIN AND MUSCLE

You can discover more information this way about cold and heat conditions, deficiencies and excesses, swelling and edema, etc.

Remember that as far as temperature of the skin goes, the surface temperature can be affected by exterior conditions. You may need to rest your hands on the skin for 15 seconds or so to get the underlying temperature.

Also, you can usually feel the temperature better with the back of your hand than with your palm or palmar side of your fingers.

Skin feels...	Means...
Cold	Possible interior cold. You may have to rest your hands on the skin for 15 seconds or so to get the feel of the underlying temperature.
Hot	<ul><li>Exterior heat: Hot on the initial touch, but heat dissipates if you keep your hands on longer.</li><li>Interior/deficient heat: Not hot on initial touch, but quite apparent when you keep your hands on longer. This is a Yin Xu heat.</li></ul>

Deficiency	You will feel the clammy sweat on the skin. If patients have deficiency, touch feels good, especially in the area or channel with the deficiency. This is always mitigated in patients who have a history of abuse or assault – they might hate touch even with a deficiency.
Excess	You will feel no sweating at all on the skin. They will also feel more uncomfortable with touch because an excess is already a condition of too much. Adding touch makes even more excess for them.
Moisture/dryness	Dry skin indicates that Body Fluids are impaired in some way. Could be a Body Fluid deficiency or blockage or Blood stasis
Swelling	• Fluid Edema: This is swelling due to fluid buildup. You will see pitting edema that is slow to refill. Can even take *minutes* to refill the divot you leave when you press on the lower leg or foot. • Qi Edema: Qi edema is a buildup of Qi at the surface. Looks a lot like fluid edema, but doesn't pit. You press down and the area refills quickly.

PALPATING HANDS AND FEET

Use the back of your hand (the dorsum) for better heat/cold detection.

Hands/Feet feel	Indicates…
Cold hands and feet	Interior cold. Could be a Yang Xu cold or a Yin excess cold.
Hot hands and feet	Interior heat. Could be a Yang excess heat or a Yin xu heat.

Heat mostly in the palms	Heat.
Heat mostly on the dorsum of the hand	Exterior heat.

PALPATING THE CHEST AND ABDOMEN

As I indicated before, there a bunch of way to do this and a lot of interpretations as to what you feel. I'm just going to give you two things to palpate for at this time. You can learn more about this later on.

Apical pulse

Called "xu li" in Chinese, this refers to the pulse of the heart itself and this is the information you are looking for with this palpation method.

The Apical pulse is found in the 5th intercostal space. Use the bulky muscle on the lateral margin of your hand, just proximal to the 5th/little finger to feel for this pulse.

Pattern	What that will feel like at the apical pulse
Normal	Should feel clear, not hard, regular beat and slow. You are feeling the Zhong Qi, or the apex of the heart. More specifically, you are feeling the pulse in the ventricle areas, especially the left ventrical where the strongest pulse is.
Zhong Qi xu	Pulse will feel weak, indicating that the Pectoral Qi is weak.
Zhong Qi leaking	The body is unable to contain and use the Zhong Qi effectively. Feels too strong, too ampy, maybe even bounding and irregular. This indicates that the Zhong Qi is leaking out. If it is severe, the Heart Qi is leaving and the Zhong Qi is almost exhausted.

PALPATING THE CHEST/HYPOCHRONDRIA

In this case, you are looking for information about the Heart, Lung, and Liver.

Presentation	Discussion
Hypochondriac area distention and pain	Indicates Lv Qi stagnation with Blood stasis. Cirrhosis and cancer of the liver can feel this way. Could be an enlarged liver for a variety of reasons. Hep C is one of them.
Palpation around rib line causes pt pain, hurts to inhale while you are palpating	If you press down the mid-clavicle line, traveling from rib to rib, patient is breathing normally and then they stop when you are around the Gallbladder level because it hurts, indicates inflammation in the Gallbladder.
Palpating on the chest, patient has distention and discomfort, touch feels worse	Phlegm/damp retention in the chest, possibly Heart and/or Lung. This is an indication the Qi cannot move freely.

ABDOMINAL PALPATION AND PAIN

First, let me say that you need to be conversant about acute conditions that affect the abdomen because these can be life-threatening. Luckily or you, in most of these the abdomen will have a hard feel to it and it will be painful upon palpation.

You'll learn far more about this in your biomedical and other classes. Not to worry. Here are a few to start you off.

Biomedical categorizations about abdominal pain

This is pain upon palpation of the areas indicated in the chart below.

Presentation	Discussion
Pain in the epigastric area	If pain present for a long time could be a gastric ulcer.
Pain in the upper hypochondriac area	Acute pain can be a perforation or stones/sludge in the Gallbladder. Feel for a wiry pulse to help confirm this.
Pain in left hypochondriac area	Possibly acute pancreatitis. Will usually have diarrhea with this.
Lower abdominal pain	Possibly uterine or ovarian problems.
Pain in lower right quadrant	Possibly appendicitis (This is considered to be an internal or intestinal carbuncle in TCM speak.)

Chinese medical categorizations about abdominal pain and palpation

We palpate for more than just pain.

Problem	Presentation and discussion
Cold	Same 'rules' as palpating the skin and muscle. Follow the link to see more.
Heat	
Deficiency	
Excess	
Swollen abdomen	• Gas and bloating This is an even swelling over the whole abdomen. • Water retention An uneven swelling in the abdomen and feels like a sack of water when you press on it. Kind of like an old school waterbed. Water retention can indicate cirrhosis. Qi deficiency can also cause this.

Diagnostics of Chinese Medicine: The Four Diagnostic Skills

Masses felt in the body and abdomen Also called Ji Ju in Chinese	• Ji or Zhen Clear shaped mass that does not move. Pain is also fixed. This is a Blood stasis problem. Hernias can be Blood stasis or phlegm retention. • Ju or Jia Doesn't have a clearly defined margin, isn't always present, not always in the same place. Pain will move around too. This is a Qi stagnation problem. Move the Qi.

BONUS SECTION:
Study Questions and Answers

What is the definition of Diagnosis in TCM?
General judgment regarding disease or syndrome as well as state of health of body by collecting and analyzing clinical materials on the basis it its' diagnostic methods.

What are the 4 Diagnostic Skills?
1. Observation/inspection
2. Listening and smelling
3. Asking
4. Feeling pulse and palpating body

What is the content you are looking for in observing/inspecting your patient?
- Shen
- Complexion
- Body
- Excretions
- Children
- Tongue

What is meant by Shen in diagnosis?
Overall demeanor or spirit.

What are the 3 aspects of Shen?

Embodiment	Outward manifestation of spirit in body itself—what is inside manifests outside
Vitality	Reflected in the energy of the person. Ranked from 1-10 in charts with 10=highest.
Luster	Reflected in the luster of eyes and complexion.

What are the 3 possible conditions of Shen/spirit?
1. Strong
2. Weak
3. False

What are the manifestations of a strong Shen?

Eyes	Sparkling, clear
Face	Lively, lustrous
Mental/emotional	Clear, alert mind Enthusiasm High Spirits Positive approach to life Stable personality Strong willpower Clear sense of direction in life
Physical	Keen reflexes Good energy Normal breathing Clear ringing voice Agile body movements

What are the characteristics of a weak Shen?

Eyes	Dull, without sparkle
Face	Lusterless complexion
Tongue	Without spirit, possible heart crack
Mental/emotional	Listless Lack of enthusiasm Confused thinking Possible apathy Depression Lack of willpower Confusion about life path Slow intellect
Physical	Shallow breathing Weak voice Slow body movement

What is False Shen?
   An extremely dangerous condition appearing during a severe chronic disease. Described as the last rays of the sun. Indicates nearness of death. Yin can no longer hold Yang, which floats upward and reddens the cheeks (like painted on surface)
Occurs very suddenly.

What are the signs of False Shen?

Sudden onset of vigor	Clear look in the eyes
Incessant talking	Wants to meet with family
Complexion reddens, but red is on surface like make-up or like it's been painted on due to the separation of Yin and Yang, resulting in Yang floating upward	Suddenly improved appetite

Name 5 ways to classify body shape
   1. Yin and Yang
   2. Five elements
   3. Prenatal and postnatal influence
   4. Body build
   5. Pain and drug tolerance

What are the 4 classifications of body shape according to Yin/Yang classification?
   1. Yang excess
   2. Yin excess
   3. Yang deficiency
   4. Yin deficiency

Yang Excess Body Type Questions

Q	A
What are the facial characteristics of a Yang Excess body type?	Tendency to red face
What kind of temperature characteristics would a Yang	• Preference for cold • Intolerance for heat

Excess type have?	• Preference for light clothing
What kind of body build would a Yang Excess type display?	Strong body build
Describe the speech mannerisms of a Yang Excess type person.	Loud voice, talkative nature
How does a Yang Excess person carry themselves when walking?	Walk with stomach and chest projecting forward
Describe the outward emotional demeanor of a Yang Excess type person.	Active, lively, tendency to laugh, high achiever.

Yin Excess Body Type Questions

Q	A
What is the facial complexion of a Yin Excess type?	Relatively dark complexion
What temperature characteristics does a Yin Excess type person have?	Preference for heat, likes to wrap up, prefers the summer and warm seasons.
What physical/body tendencies does a Yin Excess type person display?	• Tendency to obesity • Loose muscle with thick skin
Describe the general outward emotional demeanor of a Yin Excess type person.	Quiet, reticent, introverted

Yang Deficient Body Type Questions

Q	A
Describe the face of a Yang Deficient type person.	Pale or pale/bluish complexion
What kind of temperature tendencies does a Yang Deficient person display?	• Prefers warmth and has a desire to wrap up. • Has an aversion to cold and suffers from cold limbs.

What are the body characteristic tendencies of a Yang Deficient person?	• Overweight, swollen body type with weak, loose muscles. • Slow movements.
What emotional/outward demeanor would a Yang Deficient person typically display?	Low spirit with no energy or fire.

Yin Deficient Body Type Questions

Q	A
Describe the face of a Yin Deficient body type	Red cheeks and lips (sometimes), with a restless look in the eyes.
What kind of temperature tendencies does a Yin Deficient person display?	Feelings of heat
What does a Yin Deficient body look like?	Thin body, probably tall. Long shaped head, narrow shoulders, with a long flat chest.
How does a Yin Deficient body tend to stand?	Bent forward when standing or walking
How does a Yin Deficient body tend to move?	Quickly

Describe the dominant complexion colors per the Five Element classification of bodies for each of the following:

Element	Coloration
Wood	Green
Fire	Red
Earth	Yellow
Metal	Pale
Water	Dark

Definitive strong points for each of the Five Element Body Classification types:

Element	Coloration
Wood	Sinews – ropy / sinewy
Fire	Strong heart/vessels
Earth	Strong muscle system
Metal	Strong voice
Water	Strong Kidney

What is the head/face characteristic for each of the five element types?

Element	Coloration
Wood	Small head, long face
Fire	Pointed/small head
Earth	Large head with round face
Metal	Small head, square face
Water	Large head

Which of the 5 Element types has wide teeth?
    Fire

What are the 5 classification categories according to Body Build types?

Type	Tends toward…
Robust - energetic	Yang excess. Resistance to cold, suffers from hot diseases.
Compact	Smooth circulation of Qi and Blood, tends to suffer from deficiencies of Qi and Blood
Muscular	Strong Qi and Blood. Isn't easily invaded by pathogens.
Thin	Deficiency of Qi and Blood, Yin deficiency
Overweight	Qi deficiency with damp retention in the middle jiao.

If a person has facial features that look 'crammed together' with short small ears that turn outward what kind of body shape is this?
    Body shape with weak prenatal constitution

Prenatal Qi body characteristics focus on what features?
Facial features and body build – inherited body features

What about Postnatal Qi body features?
Lustre, hair, and muscle – features having to do with Qi and Blood status.

The facial complexion as a whole represents what?
Manifestation of the Heart and therefore the Shen (Mind and Spirit)

What two charactericstics does a "normal complexion" have?
Luster—bright, glowing color. Moist skin.

What is a "dominant color" in relation to complexion coloring?
- Remains the same throughout life
- Determined by race and prenatal factors
- Relates to body type.

What is a "Guest Color" in relation to complexion coloring?
Changes in dominant coloring based on work conditions, seasonal changes (which will tinge everyone slightly), environmental factors, etc.

What can you learn from complexion coloring in the clinic?
Helps determine pathology, location, nature, and prognosis for disease. This is taken in context with other diagnostic methods: observation, listening/smelling, interrogation, and feeling/palpating the body.

What is a pathological coloring?
Anything other than dominant and guest coloring is considered pathological coloring. Example: a wood type will have a greenish hue to their skin natively. They might also have a reddish tint in the summer, but a deep red would

be not a guest color, but a pathological coloring. Pale would be another example of a pathological coloring.

What is the difference between a superficial and a deep pathological color to the complexion?
- A superficial coloring indicates a mild, exterior or yang condition.
- A deep version of the same color would indicate a more severe, more internal condition affecting Yin organs.

What is indicated if a pathological color changes from deep to superficial during the course of a disease?
Indicates that the condition is getting less severe, going from deep to superficial.

What does that mean, distinct and obscure coloring?
- Distinct – bright, clear, manifesting readily
- Obscure – darkish, dull, lifeless

Both are pathological colorings, not normal.

What conditions do distinct and obscure pathological colors indicate?
- Distinct – Yang type, superficial location of pathology, Upright Qi is not exhausted.
- Obscure – Yin type of disease, located deeper in body. Upright Qi s weakened.

What is meant by Scattered and Concentrated coloring? Give the look and the meaning.
Both are pathological.
- Scattered coloring is thinly distributed and sparse. Scattered coloring indicates disease is mild, short in duration, pathogenic factors are not strong. Good prognosis

- Concentrated coloring is densely distributed and covers big bunches of skin.
  Concentrated color indicates a severe disease of long duration with strong pathogenic factors. Bad prognosis

What is meant by Thin and Thick coloring? Give the look and the meaning.
- Thin coloring: looks like a single skimpy coat of paint. Indicates a deficiency or acute disease
- Thick coloring: looks like several heavy coats of paint. Indicates an excess or chronic disease

What is meant by an abnormal/pathological Lustrous or Lusterless coloring? |Describe and give the meaning.
- Lustrous: bright, moist, vigorous, shining.
  Spirit is good, pathogens are not strong, condition is mild. Good prognosis
- Lusterless: dark, dull, gloomy, "withered".
  Spirit is weak, pathogens are strong, condition is severe Bad prognosis

What is conforming color and opposing color according to the Pattern?
- Conforming color would be the color you expect to see based on the patient's condition: example, suffer from heat and they have a reddish tinge.
- Opposing coloring would contradict the prevailing harmony

Why might a patient display opposing coloring, contradicting the prevailing disharmony you'd expect? 4 reasons.
- May be suffering from several different patterns and the complexion color reflects one of them.

- Can be influenced by the season. For example, might have a Spleen Qi deficiency, so you'd expect yellow, but it's summer, so they look reddish.
- Reflects the state of mind and spirit…if that overrides, might change coloring.
- False' complexion color—total separation of Yin/Yang, so Yang floats upward.

What is meant by "conforming" color according to the Five Elements?

When the patient's coloring doesn't match up to their condition (based on other diagnostic methods: look/observe, interrogate, listen/smell, feel/palpate); you look at the color and notice it is the "mother" color of the disharmony. Example: A patient suffers from a Liver pattern (you'd expect green), but the complexion color is dark (Water, the mother element for Wood).

What is the "slightly opposing" color according to the Five Elements?

This is the 'child' color as compared to the prevailing disharmony.
Example: A patient suffers from a Liver pattern (you'd expect green), but the complexion color is red (Fire, the child element for Wood).

What is the "opposing" color according to the Five Elements?
This is the color of the element that is the checked/overcontrolled element (element overacted upon in the control cycle) as compared to the prevailing disharmony.
Example: A patient suffers from a Liver pattern (you'd expect green), but the complexion color is yellow (Earth, the element Wood controls).

What is the "strongly opposing" color according to the Five Elements?

This is the color of the counter-checked/insulting element (the element in the control cycle that would be the controlling element as compared to the prevailing disharmony).

Example: A patient suffers from a Liver pattern (you'd expect green), but the complexion color is pale (Metal, the controlling element for Wood).

Give all conforming/opposing colors and their prognosis

Mother color conforming	Good prognosis
Son color slightly opposing	Prognosis is not so bad
Checked/overcontrol element opposing	Bad prognosis
Counterchecked/insulting color strongly opposing	Prognosis is very bad.

Four characteristics of normal complexion coloring?
- Luster
- Subtle slightly reddish hue
- "Contained" or "Veiled" color
- Moisture

A white pathological complexion color is generally indicative of what?

Xu (of qi, xue, and/or yang) and cold

Bright white	Yang deficiency
Dull white	Severe Yang xu
Pale white	Qi xu
Sallow white	Blood xu
Bluish white	Cold, especially due to Yang xu

A sallow pathological complexion color is generally indicative of what and is caused by what?

> Xu and/or dampness. Looks pale, yellowish, without luster. Can be Spleen Qi def + dampness, Kidney yang deficiency, or Blood stasis (sallow greyish)

Give the pathologies of the following shades of yellow coloring

Pale yellow	Sp Qi xu, Blood xu (anemia)
Greyish yellow	Sp Qi xu + Stagnation of Lv Qi or Blood
Dry yellow	full or empty heat in Stomach and Spleen
Ash-like yellow	Dampness
Rich yellow	Qi and blood deficiency w/dampness
Bright yellow	Jaundice—damp heat variety (yang huang)
Dark yellow	Jaundice – damp cold variety (yin huang)

Give the pathologies of the following shades of red coloring

Red cheeks	Full heat in Ht, Lu, Lv, St
Red cheekbones	Empty heat in Kid, Lu, Ht, St Blood deficiency
Floating red	Empty heat False heat/true cold

What four general conditions are indicated by a bluish/greenish complexion?
1. Cold
2. Pain
3. Blood stasis
4. Inner wind

Give the pathologies reflected in the following blue/green complexions

Pale bluish under eyes	Liver Qi stagnation
Dark bluish under eyes	Cold in Liver channel
White bluish	Cold or chronic pain
Bluish (in children)	Liver wind
Green w/red tinge	Lesser Yang syndrome
Green w/red eyes	Liver fire
Yellow-greenish cheeks	Phlegm with Liver Yang

Green nose	Stagnation of Qi with pain in abdomen
Dark reddish-green	Stagnation of Liver Qi turning to heat
Grass-like green	Collapse of Liver Qi

What 4 general states does a dark complexion color indicate?
1. Kidney xu
2. cold
3. blood stasis
4. phlegm-fluid retention

What pathologies do the following specific dark complexion colorings indicate?

Dark and dry	Ki Yin xu
Dull dark	Ki Yang xu with internal
Dark around eye sockets	• Kidney def with phlegn-fluids • Cold-dampness in lower Jiao
Dull dark, like soot	• Damp cold • Phlegm fluid retention
Faint dark	• Damp cold • Phlegm fluid retention
Very dark	Blood stasis – very severe.

General condition that a purplish complexion indicates
   Stasis

What pathologies do the following specific purple complexion colorings indicate?

Reddish purple	Blood stasis
Bluish purple	• Internal cold leading to blood • Poisoning

Give the coloring for the following emotions

Anger	green (cheeks, under eyes)
Excessive joy	red cheekbones
Worry	grayish, no luster
Pensiveness	sallow-yellow
Fear	bright white (cheeks, forehead)
Shock	bright white, bluish

Hatred	dull greenish, no luster
Craving	reddish (cheeks)
Guilt	dark, ruddy
Sadness	bluish/greenish
Grief	dark, but whitish

All different kinds of wind are related to dysfunction of what Organ?
Liver

What causes tremors?
Both internal and external wind.

Parkinson's disease and epilepsy are manifestations of what?
Internal wind

Bell's palsy is a manifestation of what?
External wind

Two reasons wind affect the body?
- Extreme heat generating wind.
  Anger, chronic depression, liver qi stagnation
- Blood deficiency
  chronic malnutrition, for example.

What is the most important sign of Wind affecting the body?
Tremors (shaking back and forth) of the head.

What does a tremor of large amplitude indicate?
A Full Wind condition, excess and/or acute in nature, generally of Liver fire or Liver yang rising. Generally short duration.

A mild tremor is indicative of what?
An Empty Wind condition--Deficiency, usually chronic, of Liver and Kidney yin. Can also be Liver-Blood deficiency. Generally longer duration.

Hypertension is tied to what kind of wind?
   Empty wind

Neck rigidity/stiffness meaning

Neck stiffness +	= ?
Aversion to wind, floating pulse	Wind invasion
Pain	Cold invasion
Slight rigidity with dizziness	Bladder and Kidney xu

Which kind of facial paralysis is CNS based and which is peripheral? Which is internal wind, which is external?

Central Nervous System	Internal wind	CVA or stroke. Very poor prognosis
Peripheral NS	External wind	Bell's Palsy Better prognosis

What are the signs of facial paralysis on the healthy side and on the affected side?

Healthy side	Affectation
• Mouth	Pulled to healthy side
• Nasolabial groove	Deep nasolabial groove
• Forehead	Can still wrinkle
Affected side	**Affectation**
• Eye	Inability to close or open the eye completely in the affected side. Tends to leak. Might turn upward
• Cheeks	Difficult to grimace, to bulge cheeks in affected side.
• Nasolabial groove	No nasolabial groove or less groove
• Forehead	Can't wrinkle forehead (CNS, not Bells)
• Mouth	Droops. Can chew, but can't get food out of this side.

Signs and symptoms of Bell's Palsy
- Flat forehead only on affected side (can wrinkle eyebrow on other)
- Can't totally close one eye (affected side) and it will leak
- Can't move muscles on affected side.
- Mouth deviates toward healthy side.

What is the underlying cause of a facial tic?
Wind

What are some limb and body signs of Wind problems?

Paralysis	Tremors or spasticity of limbs Tremors of hands and feet
Muscle twitching	Hemiplegia (paralysis or weakness on one side of body)
Contraction of the limbs	Contraction of fingers.
Opisthotonos (severe spasm in which the spine arches backward and the neck does too. Can happen in tetanus so severely that the head and heels touch. Ouch)	

Give the specific condition causing each of the following head/face/hair symptoms of Wind.

Manifestion	Meaning
Dry scalp	Lv/Ki Yin xu
Red/painful scalp	Wind heat or liver fire
Tremor of head	Lv wind
Swelling of head and face	Wind heat or toxicity
Boils and ulcers	Full or toxic heat
Head leaning to one side	Spleen or marrow xu
Head tilted, eyes rolled up	Lv wind
Late closure of fontanelles on babies	Essence xu

Give the specific condition causing each of the following facial symptoms of Wind.

Manifestion	Meaning
Acute edema	Wind-water in Lu, sudden onset.
Chronic edema	Lu and/or Sp yang Xu (Pale in color)
Acute swelling/ redness	Wind toxic-heat
Ulcers under zygomatic arch	Toxic heat in ST
Papules on nose/face	Lung heat at the Qi level
Macules on face	Blood heat
Lined face with uneven skin surface	Blood def or Heat and dryness
Deviation of eye/mouth	Wind – internal or external

Hair is a surplus of what?
  Blood

Hair falling out is a sign of what in Chinese medicine?
  Blood disorder of some kind.

What five things can cause hair to fall out?
  1. Liver blood or Kidney essence deficiency
  2. Blood heat from Liver fire
  3. Serious acute disease
  4. Chronic, protracted disease
  5. Chemotherapy or radiation

What is Alopecia?
  Hair falling out in clumps

What 3 things can cause alopecia?
  • Blood heat
  • Internal wind (will be accompanied by giddiness and wiry pulse)
  • Blood stasis (will be accompanied by dark complexion and purple tongue)

What general conditions cause dry or brittle hair?
   Blood or Yin Xu

What 4 specific conditions can cause dry or brittle hair?
   - Liver blood/Kidney essence deficiency
   - General Qi and blood deficiency
   - Spleen/Stomach deficiency
   - Chronic loss of blood

What causes greasy hair?
   Damp of phlegm

Premature graying of the hair is caused by what 4 conditions?
   - Liver blood/Kidney essence deficiency
   - General Qi and blood deficiency
   - Liver and heart fire
   - Heredity

Dandruff is caused by what three general conditions?
   - Wind
   - Xu
   - Excess

Dandruff is specifically caused by what 4 Liver conditions related to wind?
   - Liver blood def
   - Liver wind
   - Liver fire
   - Damp heat in the Liver

What is the Five Wheel Theory?
   A microsystem in which the 5 elements and their corresponding Organs are seen in the eye.

What parts of they eye reflect this Five Wheel Theory?

Part of the eye	Represents...
Iris	Wind and Liver
Canthi	Blood and Heart
Eyelids	Muscle and Spleen
Sclera	Qi and Lung
Pupil	Kidney and Water

What 4 things should you look for when observing the eye?
- Luster
- Control of the eyes
- Coloring of the eyes
- Pathological signs

What 4 channels influence the Nose?
- Main and muscle channel of LI
- Stomach channel (cnx to nose)
- Bladder muscle channel (to bridge)
- Governing vessel (flows down thru nose)

Relationship between the nose and internal organs

Area of nose	Represents...
Between the brows	Lung
Between canthi at root of nose	Heart
Bridge of nose	Liver
Sides of bridge of nose	Gallbladder
Tip of nose	Spleen
Sides of nose	Stomach

What things should you look for when observing the nose?
- Abnormal coloring
- Swelling
- Flapping alae nasi
- Nose bleeds
- Polyps
- Ulcers
- Papules

What 2 organs are reflected in the Philtrum?

- Urinary bladder (upper area of philtrum)
- Uterus and genital area (lower area of philtrum)

What do drooping lips indicate?
Spleen Qi xu

What channels influence the mouth and lips?
- LI
- Stomach
- Liver
- Heart
- Kidney
- Chong/directing,
- Du/penetrating

What aspects should you look for in mouth/lip observation?
- Abnormal coloring
- Dry or cracked lips
- Peeling lips
- Swollen lips
- Trembling lips
- Inverted lips
- Drooping lips
- Cold sores
- Mouth ulcers
- Deviation of mouth/dribbling—see stroke section

What organs do the upper and lower gums display?
- Upper gums – Stomach
- Lower gums – Large Intestine

Where is the condition of the Kidney and the Du vessel most evident in the mouth area?
Teeth and gums

What things should you look for when observing mouth?
- Tooth cavities
- Loose teeth (kidney)
- Plaque
- Teeth color

Give the root of the problem for the following specific gum problems

Gum problem	Interpretation/s
Inflammation	- Full or empty heat in ST or LI - Yin Xu
Bleeding	- Weak SP Qi not holding Blood - Empty heat in ST or KI
Bleeding, red/swollen	- Stomach fire
Receding gums	- Qi/blood xu - Stomach fire - Ki Yin xu with empty heat
Gums oozing pus – acute	- Stomach fire
Gums oozing pus - chronic	- Severe deficiency of Qi and/or Blood

What are abnormal colors for the gums?
- Pale (deficiency or cold)
- Red (Heat—empty or full)
- Purple (Stasis)

Channels that influence or enter the ears
- Gallbladder
- San Jiao
- Small Intestine
- Urinary Bladder
- Stomach
- Large Intestine connecting channel

Aspects to look for in ear observation

- Size: most important in clinic. Large is good, but should be proportional. Small is unlucky, bad, poor constitution
- Swollen – can be dampness
- Contracted ears
- Dry/contracted helix
- Sores
- Warts
- Abnormal color
- Distended blood vessels
- Excessive wax prod
- Discharge

What 3 things are nail surface abnormalities related to?
    Liver, Blood, Deficiency

Nail lunulae reflects the state of what?
    Yin and Essence

What causes the following abnormal nailbed coloring?

Nailbed discoloration	Interpretation/s
White spots	- Qi xu
Pale white nails	- Blood xu of Lv or Sp
Dull white	- Spleen or Ki Yang xu
Red	- Heat – usually full heat
Yellow	- Damp heat
Bluish	- Blood xu with internal cold
Greenish	- Severe Sp qi xu with wind
Blue/green	- Blood stasis
Dark	- Ki Yin xu - Ki Yang xu - Blood stasis
Purple and red-purple	- Lv Blood stasis
Red purple (in febrile disease)	- Blood heat

A protruding chest can be a sign of:
    Lv Qi stagnation and/or chronic retention of phlegm

A sunken chest signifies what 3 possible causes?
1. Lung Qi
2. Yin Xu
3. Kidney Xu

What 2 kinds of Edema can the 4 limbs have and how do they differ?

Type of edema	Interpretation/s
Pitting	• Phlegm/fluid retention Deficiency related
Non-pitting	• Qi stagnation More excess related

What are the 4 key points in observing secretions?
1. Amount
2. Color
3. Property
4. Smell

Describe characteristics and causes for each of the following skin conditions.

Condition	Presentation	Interpretation
Carbuncle	Swollen, red, large, painful	Heat – usually Yang excess
Furuncle	Shallow, superficial, small, round	Damp heat
Nail-like boil	Small tight millet grain look at first, then tight root with pus on top	Toxic fire
Gangrene	Dark, necrotic tissue	Yin condition. No nutrition, blood flow, O2

What is the primary means of observation for children under 3?
Index finger venule diagnosis – vein and interphalangeal joint creases.

What do the proximal, middle, and distal segments of the index finger represent in children?

Segment	Name of gate	Interpretation
Proximal	Wind gate	Less severe conditions
Middle	Qi gate	More severe condition
Distal	Life gate	Life threatening conditions

What coloring of the venule is normal in finger observation in children?
    Slightly red, perhaps a little yellow. Located inside of wind gate.

What do the following abnormal colorations in the venule represent in children?

Venule color	Interpretation/s
Purple and red	Interior heat – different from adults!
Purple and dark/black	Collateral is blocked, Blood stasis
Bright red vein	Exterior problem – different from adults!!

What does a superficial vein with a floating pulse on an index finger signify in a child?
    Common cold

What other things can you look for in kids besides finger?
- Complexion
- Orifices
- Body movements
- Spinal muscles
- Root of nose

Distention of the epigastrum and lower ab is indicative of?
    Liver Qi stagnation

Distention of abdomen with bowel problems?
    Qi stagnation in the Intestines

Slight chronic abdominal distention?
    Spleen deficiency

Severe abdominal distention indicates…?
    Damp-phlegm in LJ, edema of abdomen.

Things to do/know prior to observing the tongue?
- Arrange natural lighting (or halogen bulb in table lamp)
- What you eat can change the color of the tongue
  Examples:
    o Blueberry colors purple
    o Spicy foods can make tongue red
- Medications can change tongue color, remove coating
- Some people scrape the tongue.

What about the tongue do you observe first?
- Tongue body color
- Tongue body shape
- Tongue coating
- Veins under tongue

What are the characteristics of a normal tongue?

Aspect	Should be…
Color	Light red with luster
Movement	Flexible, supple
Moistness	Moist
Coating color	White
Coating thickness	Thin
Sublingual vessels	Light purple, not curvy/wiggle

What are the pathological colors a tongue body can be, what do they indicate?

Color	Indication/s
Pale	1. Qi deficiency 2. Yang deficiency 3. Blood deficiency 4. Cold

Red and Deep Red	• Excessive/full Heat brighter red • Deficient/empty Heat thinner body, lighter coating, possibly cracking. • If very severe, deep red in color.
Purple	All over or in spots. Indicates blood stasis or stagnation. Under-tongue veins indicate blood stasis too - dark purple, bulging, too large, curving. Caused by either Cold or Heat. • Cold: tongue will be moist, pale bluish-purple • Heat: tongue will be dry, more reddish-purple

What 4 conditions does a pale tongue body indicate?
1. Qi deficiency
2. Blood deficiency
3. Yang deficiency
4. Cold

What does a red tongue body indicate? How about deep red?

Red	Indicates heat, either full or empty. Empty heat indicated by thinner tongue body, cracking, light coating Full heat indicated by bright red.
Deep red	Severe deficient heat

What color is a Blood stasis tongue body?
Purple – perhaps all over, perhaps in spots (indicating location of stasis/stagnation). Can be due to cold or to heat. If due to cold, will be moister than drier. Will also be pale and purplish blue. If due to heat burning up body fluids/blood, will be drier and more reddish purple.

Will also probably have dark purple or blackish veins under tongue that are maybe distended or thick.

Certain nationalities and ethnic groups have purple or purple spots as a normal condition and that this does not indicate stasis.

What does a thin tongue indicate?
Yin Deficiency
(thirsty, hot flashes, sweat at night, palm heat may go with this)

Two basic conditions causing a swollen tongue and what are they?
1. Spleen Qi deficiency + damp retention. Teeth marks are likely
2. Yang Excess/excessive heat (swollen + red)

What does it mean when a tongue has cracks or fissures (4 possible indications)?
- Yin deficiency.
  If also have a heart line crack, is a Heart Yin Xu.
  May also have dryness and/or little coating.
- Blood xu with heat
- Excessive heat – hurts yin and body fluids and can cause cracking.
- Hereditary and thus no pathology

What is a heart crack and what does it mean?
A heart crack goes from the root to the tip and indicates heart yin deficiency

Describe 3 tongue cracks symptoms of Yin Deficiency.
- heart cracks – from top to bottom = heart yin def
- dryness – cracks from dryness
- cracked with little coating = yin deficiency

Blood deficiency with heat manifests as what tongue feature?
Tongue cracks

How does excessive heat cause tongue cracking?
   Damages yin and body fluids

Spleen qi deficiency with damp retention causes what tongue symptoms?
   Swollen tongue, probably with teeth marks and probably pale.

A deviated tongue means what?
   Wind stroke or other wind symptom

List 3 things that cause involuntary tongue movement
   - Tremors/wind (larger modulations)
   - Spleen qi/blood deficiency (quivering)
   - Patient held tongue out too long during tongue diagnosis!

What are prickles?
   Red spots indicating heat. Location of prickles indicates area where heat is.

What can you tell from the sublingual veins?
   Location of Blood stasis

What does a pale swollen tongue with a thin white coat and a reddish tip mean?
   Spleen qi deficiency with damp retention, mostly exterior.

Tongue presentation	Indication/s
Pale	- Qi xu - Yang xu - Blood xu - Cold
Swollen	- Damp retention - Heat
Thin coating	- Yin xu - Blood and/or Qi xu

White coating	• Normal • Cold
Reddish tip	• Heart heat

What is the normal tongue body color and coat?
  Light red body color with a thin white coat.

A yellow coating always indicates…?
  Heat
  Unless it's a false coating from coffee….

What does a greasy tongue coating look like?
  Can see individual papillae, looks like butter dried onto the tips of toothbrush bristles. Cannot scrape it off.

What do the following greasy tongue coatings represent?

Tongue presentation	Indication/s
Greasy	• Dampness
Greasy white coat	• Damp + cold
Greasy yellow	• Damp + heat. If damp is more will look greasy If heat is more, drier looking

What is the clinical difference between thin and thick coatings?
  In exterior conditions/diseases the tongue coating will be thin, indicating the disease is more on the surface of the body. If the tongue coating is thick, this indicates the disease is moving from the exterior to the inside or is already in the interior of the body.

How would a condition of heat hurting body fluids show in a tongue coating?
  Thick, somewhat dry, yellow, greasy coating.

What causes a black tongue coating?
  Extreme heat (body is red) or extreme cold (body is pale).

Diagnostics of Chinese Medicine: The Four Diagnostic Skills

What is the tongue/breath symptomatology indicating food retention?
   Curd/Tofu/Moldy coating—thick, lumpy, scrapes off easily. Also, breath is sour.

What is the difference between a greasy tongue coating and a tofu/curdy/mouldy tongue coating?
   Greasy is finer and smoother, can see the individual papillae, hard to scrape off. Tofu-like coating is thicker, lumpier/rougher, can't see papillae and scrapes off easily.

How do you tell what color the tongue body is when the coat is too thick to see through?
   Look at the tip and the sides.

Draw/describe the tongue map
   Overall, the tongue represents the heart. However:

Tongue part	Reflects health of...
Sides	• Liver and Gallbladder
Tip	• Heart
Arc just behind tip	• Lungs
Center 1/3 of tongue	• Stomach and Spleen
Back 1/3 of tongue	• Lower Jiao • Kidney • Bladder

What is the definition of a peeled coat? Exfoliated? Map? Mirror?

Presentation	Interpretations
Peeled	Bald in spots
Exfoliated	Bald in smaller spots than in peeling
Map coating	Bald in bigger spots, very defined edges
Mirror coat	No coating left

What do these coatings mean?
   Yin deficiency in organs indicated by the location of the peel/exfoliation/map coating on the tongue

What is a mirror coat and what is the significance?
   A mirror coating on a tongue is no coating at all.
   Indication: severe Stomach Qi and Yin deficiency.

Describe the significance of the following coating colors:

Color	Interpretations
White	• Normal • Cold
Yellow	• Heat Interior or Exterior
Grey	Process between white and black • Cold – pale body • Heat – red body • Internal syndrome
Black	• Extreme heat – red body • Extreme cold – pale body

What are true and false coatings?
- True coating is the real color and condition of the coat
- False coating indicates color of coat artificially altered—foods or scraping…maybe meds too.

What do the following coating conditions indicate?

Coating or condition	Interpretations
Moist	• Normal • Cold • Damp • Healthy condition of body fluids
Dry	• Yin or body fluid consumption • Heat
Thick	• Damp or phlegm retention • Food stagnation • Interior condition with long/chronic history.
Thin	• Normal • Superficial or exterior condition • Acute/beginning of an invasion/condition
Bean Curd	• Food stagnation

		Primary indication, esp with sour breath.
	•	Damp or phlegm retention
Greasy, slippery, or sticky	•	Damp or phlegm retention Primary indication
	•	Food stagnation
Exfoliated, peeled, mapped, or mirror	•	Yin deficiency
Mirror coating	•	Stomach Qi xu
	•	Extreme Yin xu
	•	Could be both
Cracked tongue	•	Yin xu
Red, swollen body with thin white coating	•	Red = heat
	•	Swollen can be damp retention or swelling from heat
	•	Coat means isn't severe yet
Pale, cracked body with peeled coating	•	Pale = qi, yang, blood xu or cold
	•	Cracking = Yin or Body Fluid xu, Blood xu
	•	Peeled = yin xu
Red prickles all over tongue body	•	Heart heat
Red swollen tongue with red spots, cracks, thin white coating	•	Red=heat
	•	Spots = Heart heat
	•	Cracks = yin xu
	•	Coating = not too severe or too deep
Red thin body + peeling coat	•	Red = heat
	•	Thin = xu
	•	Peeling = Yin xu
Swollen, red body + greasy and peeled coat		Red + swelling = yang excess/excessive heat. Greasy coating implies damp retention. Peeled coating tells us that the yin is probably damaged by the heat and is therefore deficient.
Red tongue with cracks and a peeled coating		Red indicates heat. Cracks and peeling both indicate yin deficiency. So, yin deficiency with empty heat.
Narrow bodied tongue with a red tip and yellow, greasy		Thin/narrow tongue indicates 1) yin xu, 2) blood and qi xu Red tip and yellow coat indicate heart heat

coating?	(former) and heat in general (latter) Greasy part indicates dampness. Thin tongue most important: yin deficiency probably. Red tip: heart heat. Secondarily, some dampness and some heat.
Swelling at the tip of the tongue + red body + yellow coating	If tip only, is heart pathology. When combined with the red body (heat) and a yellow coat (also heat), then heart (excessive) heat
Pale tongue with pointed swelling at tip, cracks, and a thin white coat	Pale is qi, blood, or yang deficiency, possibly cold too. Swelling at tip in heart area indicates heart heat. Cracks could be yin, body fluid, or blood deficiency Heart heat is a good bet. Thin white coat says not too much heat everywhere, probably cracking is yin deficiency. Paleness could be blood deficiency.

A thin tongue body indicates what 3 conditions?
- Yin deficiency
- Blood deficiency
- Qi deficiency

Under what 5 conditions will a tongue body be swollen?
- Qi deficiency
- Yang deficiency
- Damp retention
- Excessive heat
- Toxicosis

Three possible causes of a flaccid tongue body
- Blood and Qi deficiency
- Extreme Blood and Qi deficiency
- Yin deficiency

Three causes of teeth marks.

- Qi deficiency
- Yang deficiency
- Dampness retention

Why would a tongue move and quiver beyond the patient's control?
  Wind

Red spots and prickles are an indication of …?
  Heat. Spots are larger and indicate more extreme heat.

What do purple spots mean (assuming the patient is not Pakistani)?
  Blood stasis

List the 10 traditional questions
  1. Aversion to cold and fever
  2. Sweating
  3. Head and Body
  4. Urine/Stool
  5. Food/drink
  6. Chest/Abdomen
  7. Deafness
  8. Thirst
  9. Previous illnesses
  10. Cause of disease

List the 16 questions (more modern)
  1. Pain
  2. Food and taste
  3. Stool and urine
  4. Thirst and drink
  5. Energy levels
  6. Head, face, body
  7. Chest and abdomen
  8. Limbs

9. Sleep
10. Sweating
11. Ears and eyes
12. Feeling of cold, heat, fever
13. Emotional symptoms
14. Sexual symptoms
15. Women's symptoms
16. Children's symptoms

Where do you see a yin edema?
On the lower body, below the waist

Where do you see yang edema?
On the upper body above the waist.

What questions should you ask first in a patient interview?
1. What is the chief complaint?
   Should be short, in the patient's words, not be a diagnosis, include length of time occurring
2. Present history
   Includes chief complaint, origination of problem, length of time occurring.
   Includes treatment tried already
   What makes it better/worse
   Current symptoms
3. Past history
   Less relations to chief complaint
4. Personal history
5. Family history

First 2 things you establish when a patient walks in?
- Observe first—walk, demeanor, body shape.
- Listen to voice, sound of breathing, coughing, etc.

What is the proper way to interrogate a patient?

- Be polite and welcoming. Never interrupt patient directly. Be open minded, don't assume.
- Discuss confidentiality
- Never talk about other patients with your patients. Don't mention pt's name or symptoms.
- Do you blindly follow the 10/16 questions?
  No. You ask logically and follow the leads.

There are 5 very important principles of interviewing. What are they?
  1. Establish patient's chief complaint
  2. Keep an open mind
  3. Ask questions logically
  4. Don't directly interrupt
  5. Don't disclose private information

What are the basic questions for Question 1 of the 10 Traditional Questions: aversion to cold and fever?
- When did it start/how long has it lasted?
- How did it start? (walking in the rain, exposure to another person with cold, etc.)
- What is the relationship of the chills/fever (both, which is more, one or the other, alternate?)?

Chills and fever review

Chills and fever	Interpretations
Simultaneous chills and fever	• Exterior syndrome
Chills greater than fever	• Wind cold invasion
Fever greater than chills	• Wind heat
Fever but no chills	• Interior heat
Chills only, no fever	• Interior cold

How do you tell if an interior cold is full or empty?
  Interior cold is chills only, no fever.

If it's empty cold (yang def) = pale/swollen tongue, swollen body, bright white face. If it's full cold (yin excess) = acute, not relieved by wrapping up.

How do you tell if interior heat is excess or deficient?
Fever only is Interior Heat.
Excessive (yang excess) : red cheeks, red tongue/yellow coat, high fever, big pulse, big thirst. Deficient (yin deficiency): red cheekbones, red tongue with cracks, thin coat, slender tongue, night sweats, tidal fevers.

What chill/fever symptom is alternating between the 2?
Malaria and/or Shaoyang syndrome

What questions do you ask about sweating?
- When do you sweat?
- Where do you sweat?
- Is it cold/hot? (nature of sweating)

Sweating review

Sweating	Interpretations
Heavy sweating during the day while moving around	• Yang xu • Qi xu
Night sweats	• Yin xu
Cold sweat	• Yang xu
Hot sweating	• Yin xu
Spontaneous, all over sweat	• Qi xu • Yang xu

What are the 4 subcategories of Exterior condition sweating?
1. external heat
2. external cold
3. external deficiency
4. external excess

Describe the 3 subcategories of internal syndrome with localized sweating.

Sweating location	Interpretations
Head only	• Upper jiao • Damp heat
Palms/soles	• Sp/St damp heat
One side of the body only	• Channel blocked on non-sweating side

What 3 questions do you ask regarding pain?
1. Where is it specifically?
2. How long have you had it?
3. What is the nature of the pain?
4. When does it occur?
5. What makes it better or worse?

What do the following types (nature) of pain indicate?

Nature of pain	Interpretations
Distending pain	• Liver Yang rising – in the case of headache • Qi stagnation
Throbbing pain	In the head, Liver yang rising
Stabbing, fixed, worse at night	Blood stasis
Dull pain	• Qi and Blood xu • Damp phlegm retention if pain is in the head.
Sharp	Excess
Moving pain	Qi stagnation
Cold or hot	Indicates cold or heat!
Heavy head with pain	Signals damp and phlegm in headaches. Can also have heavy pain in the body –can be damp/phlegm, can be Spleen qi xu.

What are the types of headaches?

Location of headache	Type of headache
Forehead	Yangming headache Stomach and Large Intestine channels

Vertex	Jueyin headache
	Liver channel at top of head
Occiput	Taiyang headach
	Bladder channel at back of head
Temples	Shaoyang headache
	Gallbladder channel goes here, as does one branch of Liver hannel
Whole head	Shaoyin headache
	Kidney channel goes here.
	Can also be Qi and Blood xu if it also feels empty

What 4 things do you need to ask about urine?
1. Color
2. Amount
3. Frequency
4. Pain

What do the following urine colors indicate?

Color	Indications
Pale yellow	Cold or deficiency
Dark yellow	Heat or excess
Bright yellow	Jaundice
Redness	Bleeding – can be excess or deficient in nature

What could the following urine amounts indicate if they are pathological?

Amount	Indication
Profuse	Deficiency - usually Yang xu
Scanty	Excess – often excess heat, can be deficient heat though.

Five causes/types of Lin syndrome
- Qi stagnation
- Blood Lin Syndrome
- Heat Lin
- Stones
- STD's

What is normal for stool?
   Brown, formed (S-shaped), floating, daily is ideal.

Three causes for a pale or white stool?
   1. Gallbladder bile secretion insufficiency
   2. Lv/Gb Qi stagnation
   3. Stones in Gb

What 8 things do you ask regarding the stool?
   1. Color
   2. Frequency
   3. Quality
   4. Odor
   5. Mucus?
   6. Body fluids?
   7. Burning?
   8. When problem occurred if any.

What can diarrhea indicate?
   - Spleen qi xu, cannot hold liquids
   - Damp heat (dysentery sx)
   - Yang deficiency, if diarrhea is chronic and occurs around 5am.

Two things to ask (subcategories) about food.
   - Food preferences and cravings
   - How's your appetite?
     o Good = normal
     o Poor = not so good.
     o Good, but eat all the time = not so good. Full or empty fire, SP/ST disharmony

What 3 things do you ask about drinking/fluid intake (not drinking alcohol)?

- Are you thirsty?

Answer	Indication
No	Could be normal. Check the tongue.
Yes	• Possibly normal but hot from being outside • Heat sign • Water retention, not going where it is supposed to

- Do you prefer to drink hot or cold?

Answer	Indication
Hot/warm/room	Can indicate internal cold
Cold	Internal heat sign

- How much water do you drink?

Answer	Indication
Lots	• Excessive internal heat • Loss of fluids • Chronic disease hurting Ki Yin, can be deficiency.
Little, doesn't want to drink	• Deficient heat due to Yin xu • Dampness – water isn't going where it should • Dry mouth and just wants to rinse mouth? Blood stasis

What two things do you ask about deafness?
1. Do you have hearing loss?
2. Do you have tinnitus?

What are your follow up questions if your patient says they have either hearing loss or tinnitus?
1. What side is it on?
2. What is the quality of the sound you hear?

What is the most common cause of total deafness?
Excess, blockage.

What does echo or hearing double indicate?
Liver wind, liver heat, kidney deficiency, lower jiao deficiency.

What do the following tastes in the mouth mean?

Taste	Indications
Bland	• No specific indication • Sp/St Qi xu
Sweet	• Sp/St damp heat
Acid regurgitation	• Heat in Lv • Heat in St
Sour	• Food stagnation
Bitter	• St heat • Gallbladder heat
Salty	• Ki xu • Cold
Metallic	• Lung • Also endocrine disorders • Medications

What questions do you ask about sleep?
- How long have problems been happening?
- More trouble going to sleep or staying asleep?
- How long do you sleep?
- Do you wake feeling rested?
- Do you dream? Is it vivid?

What are the s/sx of the following syndromes?

Syndrome	Indications
Ht/Ki disharmony	• Difficulty getting to sleep • Palpitations • Excessive dreaming • Night sweats • Lower back soreness/weakness

Ht/Sp deficiency	• Sleeping lightly, waking easily, plus…
	   o Palpitations
	   o Poor appetite
	   o Pale tongue

Food stagnation/retention	• Restless sleep with...
	   o Belching
	   o Abdominal distention

What does excessive sleeping do to the Qi?
Scatters it! This causes dampness and blocks the Spleen

What questions do you ask about menstrual cycles?
- How long has this lasted?/ When did it start?
- Is there pain and where is it?
- Is there something that causes the pain?
- Does cold/heat make it better/worse?
- Is the pain related to your period?
- Re menses: What is the color, amount, smell? Do you have clots in the bloods?
  Strong smell is excess, heat, damp heat.
  Weak smell is deficiency
  If lots are larger than a dime, this indicates stasis

What are the characteristics of each of these syndromes?

Syndrome	Characteristics
Early menstrual syndrome	• 8-9 days early • Large amount of blood
Late menstrual syndrome	• 8-9 days alte • Scanty menses, often with abdominal pain
Irregular menstrual syndrome	• Never know when it's coming.
Amenorrhea	• 3+ months without a period • Patient often pale, blood xu s/sx

Short period	• Short cycle
	• Profuse amount
	• Fresh red color
	   Excess blood heat
	• Darker red color
	   Qi xu.

What are the causes of each of these syndromes?

Syndrome	Cause
Early menstrual syndrome	• Blood heat • Qi xu
Late menstrual syndrome	• Blood xu • Cold contractions
Irregular menstrual syndrome	• Lv Qi stagnation
Amenorrhea	• Qi and Blood xu

What questions do you ask about abnormal uterine bleeding?
1. When did it start?
2. What is the reason?
3. Color?
4. Amount?
5. Clots?

What are the 3 pulse points and which fingers do you use for each of them?
- Cun is the 1st position. Index finger
- Guan is the 2nd position. Middle finger. This is located medial to the radial styloid process.
- Chi is the 3rd position. Ring finger

What is the proper finger placement to use when taking a pulse?
- Find the medial styloid point proximal to the wrist with the middle finger and go medial to it. This is the Guan position.
- Place the index finger distal to this just below or near the crease of the wrist. This is the Cun position.
- Place the ring finger proximal to the middle finger, furthest away from the wrist. This is the Chi position.

Define the location of each and the indications on either side in relation to pulse taking:

Position	Definition and indication
Cun	1st position, just below or near the crease of the wrist, distal to the radial styloid process. • Left wrist = Heart • Right wrist = Lung
Guan	2nd position, inside of the radial styloid process. • Left wrist = Liver • Right wrist = Spleen/Stomach
Chi	3rd position, distal from the wrist. • Left wrist = Ki, Ki Yin, lower abdomen, Shen • Right wrist = Ki, Ki Yang, lower abdomen, Mingmen

What are the three depths of pulses and what do you feel with each?

Depths	
Lifting	• Light touch – just at the surface • Feel for superficial pulses
Searching	• Medium pressure • Feel for shape and nature of pulse
Pressing	• Deep pressure • Feeling for root, for deep pulses

How long does TCM recommend you feel the pulse?
    50 beats

What is the best posture for the patient when you take the pulse (per TCM and for testing purpose, I mean)?
    Arm parallel to the ground, sitting comfortably, not too extended, arm on a pillow is best. Alternately, lying down is good.

What are dorsal, oblique, and flying pulses?
   Unusual pulse positions – radial artery runs obliquely over the radius instead of down the medial length of the radial bone.

How many pathological pulses are there?
   28

How many strange pulses and death pulses are there in addition to the 28 pathological pulses?
   10 strange pulses
   7 death pulses

What are the six categories of pulses?
   1. Superficial
   2. Deep
   3. Slow
   4. Rapid
   5. Deficient
   6. Excess

What speed of pulse indicates heat?
   Rapid or rapid feeling (90bpm or more)

What speed of pulse indicates cold?
   As a rule, slow. 60bpm or less.

Name the three crisis pulses
   Scattered (superficial)
   Swift (rapid)
   Minute/Feeble/Faint (deficient)

Go back and review the pulse charts in the chapter on pulse diagnosis. Definitely memorize anything that is bolded.
No need to reiterate that here.

Touching, pressing, feeling and pulse taking are all forms of palpation. What 2 things should you make sure you do prior to palpating?
- Clean your hands
- Warm your hands, especially in cold weather!

What kinds of information can you get from palpating the skin and muscle beneath it? (3 pairs of opposites plus one more single category)
- Hot/cold
- Deficient/Excess
- Dry/moist
  Condition of body fluids (moist or not)
- The one with no opposite: swelling/edema

How do you feel the difference between internal and external heat when palpating skin/muscle?
- Internal heat: not hot to touch, but can feel it if you leave your hand in place.
- External heat: hot to the touch, but not so much if you keep it there.

What does it mean when it feels better to the patient for you to touch or press on an affected area?
    Deficiency

What does it mean when it feels worse to the patient for you to touch or press on an affected area?
    Excess

What can you tell about body fluid condition by palpating the skin?
- If moist, body fluids undamaged.
- If dry, body fluids are suffering.

What is the difference between Qi and Water edemas?

- Qi edema does not leave a lasting depression when you press into it. Much faster recovery time than water edemas.
- Water edemas take a long time to spring back when you press into them.

A patient with hiccups that likes to drink hot liquids and says it feels better when you palpate her stomach. What might you ascertain her problem to be?

Hiccups + hot liquids preferred + touch me = deficiency of stomach—probably deficient cold in stomach.

Another patient comes in with hiccups. He like drinking cold beverages exclusively. He is more uncomfortable when you palpate/touch his stomach. What condition might you expect him to suffer from?

Hiccups + likes cold beverages + don't touch my tummy = excess heat in stomach.

Cold hands and feet can indicate what sort of conditions?
Internal cold, could be yin excess or yang deficiency.

Hot hands and feet?
Yang excess or yin deficiency.

Internal heat can be indicated by what temperature conditions of the hand? External heat?
- Palm heat = internal (yin side)
- Dorsal heat on hand = external (yang side)

What is the apical pulse? Where and how is it felt? And how should a normal apical pulse feel to the doc?

This is the pulse from the tip of the heart (inferior portion, points left), indicating the health of the Central/Zhong Qi. You feel it with the meaty part of the side of your hand below the pinky at the 5th intercostal space on the left.

Should feel clear, regular, slow…not hard.

What do the following pathological apical pulses tell you?

Pathology	Indication
Weak apical pulse	• Pectoral/Zhong Qi is weak, deficient
Too strong apical pulse	• Pectoral/Zhong Qi is leaking out
Bounding, irregular, flooding apical pulse	• Heart Qi is leaving • Zhong Qi is almost gone

What do the following distending pains indicate?

Pathology	Indication
Distention and pain in the hypochondria	• Liver Qi stagnation with Blood stasis • Also: Liver cancer, cirrhosis, Hep c, liver enlargement
Distention and discomfort all over the chest area with palpation	• Phlegm/damp retention in the Lung • Phlegm/damp retention in the Heart • Qi cannot move freely

The following biomedical conditions should be known by TCM docs. ….

Pathology	Indication
Very hard abdomen anywhere you palpate	• Acute abdominal syndrome. Life threatening!
Long term pain in epigastric area	• Possible stomach ulceration
Acute pain, upper right quadrant in hypochondriac area	• Gallbladder perforation or stones Feel for a wiry pulse!
Acute pain, upper left quadrant, hypochondriac area	• Acute pancreatitis Ask if they have diarrhea
Pain in lower abdominal area	• Possible uterine problems – bleeding or endometriosis • Ovarian problems, like ovarian cyst

In regards to abdominal swelling, what do these presentations mean from a Chinese medical perspective?

Pathology	Indication
Swollen abdomen, swelling is constant, does not change when patient rolls over	• Gas and bloating
Swollen abdomen, swelling moves like a water bed when patient rolls over	• Water retention in the abdominal cavity. Usually Qi deficiency causing fluid movement problems, but can also be a sign of cirrhosis.

What is the TCM terminology for abdominal masses?
Ji Ju

What are the s/sx for the two types of Ji Ju and what is the likely indication?

Ji or Zhen type s/sx	Indication
• Clearly felt margins of the mass • Unmoving • Has fixed pain	Blood stasis
Ju or Jia type s/sx	**Indication**
• No clearly defined margins • Mass is not always in the same place • Has pain that seems to move from place to place also.	Qi stagnation

About the Author

Cat Calhoun is a licensed acupuncture practitioner in the State of Texas and soon to be in the State of Florida as well. She attended AOMA Graduate School of Integrative Medicine, earning a Masters degree in Acupuncture and Oriental Medicine. She is passionate about teaching, both formally and informally. Cat has single-handedly created and managed CatsTCMNotes.com since 2008, dispensing notes and clinical pearls to students and practitioners for the past 11 years. She is also passionate about learning, and is currently in love with Master Tung's Acupuncture system.

This book, *Diagnostic Skills in Chinese Medicine: Book 1 – The Four Diagnostic Skills*, has a companion book for the 2nd half of your Diagnostics education in Chinese medicine. Look for it Amazon: *Diagnostic Skills in Chinese Medicine: Book 2 – Symptom Analysis and Syndrome Differentiation.* Both of these books are vital for framing your understanding of the diagnostic methods and skills, critical information you need in order to treat effectively in clinic. Both books are available in digital and print format.

www.ingramcontent.com/pod-product-compliance
Lightning Source LLC
Chambersburg PA
CBHW021814170526
45157CB00007B/2590